Contents

PRIMARY CARE DEVELOPMENT

Practitioners and Practices

a conflict of values?

Julian Pratt
General Practitioner, Sheffield

Foreword by **Professor Martin Roland**
Department of General Practice, Manchester

Series Editors **Pat Gordon** and **Diane Plamping**

Published in association with King's Fund, London

Radcliffe Medical Press
Oxford and New York

©1995 Julian Pratt

Radcliffe Medical Press Ltd
18 Marcham Road, Abingdon, Oxon OX14 1AA, UK

Radcliffe Medical Press, Inc.
141 Fifth Avenue, New York, NY 10010, USA

British Library Cataloguing in Publication Data

A Catalogue record for this book is available from the British Library.

ISBN 1 85775 140 X

Library of Congress Cataloging-in-Publication Data is available.

Typeset by AMA Graphics Ltd, Preston
Printed and bound in Great Britain

Series introduction

Primary care development is arguably the most important topic for the NHS to get to grips with in the rapidly changing environment of the 1990s. This new series of books about primary care development is intended to be topical, useful and, before very long, out-of-date. It is based on the current work of the King's Fund Primary Care Group and the ideas, experience and inspiration of a number of people who have worked with us and shared their enthusiasms.

Primary care is often used to mean general practice. Here it is used to mean the broader network of community-based health services which in the UK allow us to manage 90% of care outside hospitals; to manage earlier, safer discharge from hospitals, and to maintain people at home who do not want to be institutionalized.

From a position of relative neglect and invisibility, primary care has shot to the top of the NHS policy agenda. This has much to do with the NHS reforms and the drive to control public spending. Like all industrialized nations faced with ever-increasing costs in health care, we are experimenting with reorganization. Since hospitals use most NHS resources, this is where most attention was directed and primary care became the focus only as a potentially cheaper option. But the drive for efficiency and value for money coincides with other powerful influences which challenge us to examine alternatives to traditional ways of delivering services. If effective primary care really is the key to successful health services in the future, then recognizing its distinctive characteristics, and what we value about it as well as what we want to change becomes critical. In other words, primary care has development needs in its own right quite apart from the current emphasis on the shift from secondary to primary care – the so-called substitution agenda.

This new series is about ideas and services which are being developed and tested around the country. It is about work-in-progress in a period of extraordinary change. It is about general practice as well as general practitioners; about developing new kinds of primary care organizations; about the capacity to deliver high-quality nursing care at home; and about polyclinics and resource centres, specialists and generalists. The series begins, appropriately, with Julian Pratt's book on general practice. The underlying model of general practice is being challenged by new ideas of the role of the practitioner and the organization in which she works. Forthcoming titles address practice management, the fastest growing health care occupation in the UK, and new ways of extending primary care beyond family-based practice to polyclinics and hospitals at home. We hope the ideas in these books contribute to the debate about the future shape of the NHS and are useful to the people working in the middle of these major changes now.

Pat Gordon
King's Fund
London

February 1995

Foreword

The pace of change in the NHS is so great that many within primary care wonder whether the core values of general practice, which have led to Britain leading the way in the world in primary health care, can survive without being damaged beyond recognition. This book takes a unique analytical approach. Julian Pratt has drawn on three conferences organized by the King's Fund which were designed to see how the core of general practice could be maintained and strengthened in a changing world.

Dr Pratt identifies those values which are central to the practitioner for whom a one-to-one relationship with her patient is paramount. He contrasts these with the 'practice values' which are needed by a range of health professionals whose focus is how to maximize the health of a practice population within available resources. He addresses the inevitable conflicts between trying to accommodate both sets of values within one practice organization. He argues that patients will lose out if either set of values seeks to dominate. Practices need to acknowledge that a constructive tension can exist between the two approaches, and that practitioners and practices need to find ways of building on both sets of values in order to realize the full potential of primary health care. Many feel currently that if general practice as we know it survives, it will do so in spite of the organizational changes rather than because of them. This book takes a much more positive view. It recognizes the difficulties, but sets out a conceptual framework which addresses both the needs of individual patients and those of practice populations.

This book will appeal to all primary care staff – doctors, nurses, and managers in addition to those who have responsibility for developing primary care within health authorities. It should be read by anyone who is feeling depressed about the future of primary care in the NHS.

Martin Roland
Professor of General Practice
Manchester

February 1995

Acknowledgements

This book is based on a series of conferences run by the King's Fund Primary Care group during 1994. The ideas and inspiration for this book are those of the speakers at these conferences, who are listed below, and of the conference audiences who contributed to the discussions. The author thanks the speakers and other colleagues who have commented on drafts of this book for their suggestions and comments but accepts full responsibility for any errors, omissions or idiosyncratic interpretations. Thanks are also due to Paul Schatzberger for providing the photographs.

Jane Broadbent	Lecturer, Sheffield University Management School
Eleanor Brown	Practice Development and Fundholding Manager, Paxton Green Health Centre, London
Tyrrell Evans	General Practitioner, Paxton Green Health Centre, London
John Horder	Retired London GP, Past President of the Royal College of General Practitioners, Chairman of the Centre for the Advancement of Interprofessional Education

June Huntington	Fellow of the King's Fund College and Independent Consultant in Health Care Management
Linda Lamont	Director of the Patients Association
Richard Laughlin	Professor of Accounting, Sheffield University Management School
Denis Pereira Gray	Professor, Institute of General Practice, University of Exeter
Brenda Poulton	Community Nursing Adviser to the Royal College of Nursing
Belinda Pratten	Chair of Health Rights
Kieran Sweeney	Research Fellow, Institute of General Practice, University of Exeter
Martin Walsh	General Practitioner, Birley Health Centre, Sheffield

Terminology

The patient	It is never easy to find an appropriate term for 'person', who is the 'client', 'consumer', 'customer' or 'user' of the NHS. The term 'patient' is used as it is unambiguous and is capable of encompassing some of the special characteristics of a person who feels ill as well as a person dealing with a health care system.
The practitioner	Although drawing particularly on the history and experience of the general practitioner (GP), the term 'practitioner' is used to include GPs and others (including nurses and counsellors) who have one-to-one relationships with patients. For clarity, the term applies only to those employed by the practice rather than the 'primary health care team'.
Gender	Both patients and practitioners are mostly referred to as female, with the intention of including both men and women. This reflects the use of the term practitioner to include nurses,

counsellors and the increasing proportion of women GPs.

The practice
The term 'practice' refers to the organization comprising GPs and all those directly employed by them, in contrast to the individual practitioners who work in the organization.

Primary care
'Primary care' is used to describe the first point of contact of the patient with the health care services, in contrast to secondary care, which is the layer of (often hospital-based) services to which patients may be referred from primary care. In the UK, the main primary care provider organizations are general practices, community health trusts (community nursing), pharmacists, opticians, dentists and hospital accident and emergency departments.

Primary health care
Primary health care is a much broader concept than primary care, amounting to a blueprint for a new approach to health care, as described in the 1978 World Health Organization conference at Alma Ata. It is 'an approach to the provision of health services which emphasizes the *promotion* of health through a partnership between health and other professionals and the community, as well as a system of treatment and curative care based on meeting the health needs of the majority of the population to be served'[1]. It rests on the three pillars of participation, intersectoral collaboration and equity.

Abbreviations

DHA   District Health Authority

FHSA   Family Health Services Authority

FMI   Financial Management Initiative

GMSC General Medical Services Committee of the British Medical Association

GP   General Practitioner

NHS   National Health Service

RCGP Royal College of General Practitioners

Introduction

This chapter introduces the main themes that will be explored in the book and provides an outline summary of its conclusions.

There are many influences that are leading to an increased emphasis on primary care in the NHS.

- Demographic changes have increased the importance of the management of chronic illness in relation to treating acute episodes of illness.

- The development of less invasive and more effective technical procedures reduces the time patients need to stay in hospital but may increase the time during which they need care at home.

- As specialization in secondary care increases and 'general physicians' and 'general surgeons' are replaced by 'consultants with an interest in . . .', the need for a generalist primary care service increases.

- The NHS may reduce its expenditure by externalizing 'hotel' and transport costs, transferring them to patients and their families.

- Users of the NHS are expressing a preference for community-based services delivering an appropriate local service.

- Perhaps most importantly, the influence of primary care on the commissioning of secondary care has increased the power of primary care to shape the overall delivery of health care.

Primary care providers have the opportunity to play a pivotal role in the development of the NHS as a primary health care led service. This arises centrally from the change from rationing of services (allocation of resources) on the basis of the historical claims of providers (particularly in secondary care) to rationing on the basis of *local health need*, and the involvement of primary care providers (through the fundholding mechanism or non-fundholding consortia) in this process.

In order to play this role, general practice and other primary care providers will need to be different from how they have been in the past. If this change takes place without a genuine appreciation of the nature of general practice, there is a danger that some of its essential qualities may be damaged or lost.

The King's Fund London Commission proposed increasing resources for primary health care in order to:

- strengthen core general practice

- extend primary health care

- reshape the primary/secondary care boundary.

As part of its commitment to taking forward the work of the Commission, the King's Fund Primary Care Group organized a series of 'Capital Conferences' around each of these three themes. This book, on the theme of identifying and strengthening core general practice, is derived from the presentations, formal discussions and informal conversations that occurred at the conferences. The focus of the conferences on the *values* and *role* rather than the *tasks* of general practice is reflected in this book, the purpose of which is to contribute to an improved understanding of general practice, both by those who work in it and by those who commission and use its services.

The conferences chose to focus on the values of general practice, rather than more narrowly on the values of GPs or more widely on the values of primary health care. In particular, community health trusts and their community nurses have thus not been directly considered, in spite of their importance as providers of primary health care and their close working relationships with general practice. It seems likely that the core values of community nursing have much in common with those of general practice. This book may provide a framework for exploring the values of others providing primary health care – both as individuals and in organizations.

General practice is a cornerstone of primary care in this country. The traditional model has been challenged by new visions of its role, particularly a responsibility for improving health as well as for the care of illness, and a responsibility for populations as well as for individuals. The past independence of general practitioners has allowed innovation and good practice to flourish but has also resulted in some unacceptably poor practice[2]. The failure of the medical profession to address this problem has resulted in this challenge being taken up by NHS management, through the Family Health Services Authorities (FHSAs) and health commissions.

There is low morale among many general practitioners, and the most commonly expressed reasons given for dissatisfaction are practical ones, such as the amount of paperwork, the clinical work-load (especially out of hours) and interaction with administrators[3]. There is also a debate within general practice about the 'task of the new general practitioner'[4]. It seems likely that the low morale is in part related to the uncertainty about the changing tasks and, even more fundamentally, the changing underlying values and role of general practice. There is a feeling among many GPs that their core values are being eroded and that the good general practitioner now survives in spite of, rather than because of, the organizational context.

A *core value* of general practice is a very broad, high-level characteristic or quality, which is both wanted by those who use the service and needed in the judgement of those who provide it. It is a characteristic that is prized and without which the service is lacking something of importance. It is derived from past experience and transmitted to the future, much as the essence of an organism is transmitted by its genetic material.

The aim of the Capital Conferences was, therefore, to:

- examine the way in which current developments may be altering the core values and content of general practice

- clarify the nature of this core

- nourish the core without colluding with the avoidance of change.

There has been an historical development from the practitioner as a doctor working alone or with a small group of colleagues, to the practice as an organization. The values identified as being at the core of general practice appeared to fall into two broad groups.

- The first group, described here as *practitioner* values, are those appropriate to the one-to-one relationship with a patient. These are the values of doctors, nurses and counsellors. They reflect the central importance of the individual patient and the need for the practitioner to give the highest priority to that individual.

- The second group, described here as *practice* values, are those appropriate to improving the health of a population. These are the values of practice managers, some doctors and nurses, and colleagues outside the practice, from health commissions to ministers of state. They reflect the central importance of maximizing health gain for a population within the available resources.

Traditionally, a general practice used to share the values of its practitioners, that is to say the focus on the individual patient. What I have called practice values were held not within the general practice but by health authorities and the NHS management structure. Since the 1960s, many general practices, with the encouragement of the Royal College of General Practitioners, have taken on practice values. Since the 1990 contract, these values, particularly those related to the allocation of resources, have had an impact on *all* general practices.

Just as doctors in general practice have experienced uncertainty about their core values, similar dilemmas have arisen for others working in primary care, in particular practice nurses. Many have been recruited primarily to meet the needs of the practice (eg to achieve population targets and run well-person clinics). They thus need to subscribe to the core values of the practice, yet from their past experience of one-to-one patient care, nurses will also have brought a set of core values that are referred to here as the values of the practitioner rather than of the practice.

These two sets of values in some ways support each other but in other ways are in conflict. Many general practices have found ways of accommodating both sets of values without making them explicit, but this accommodation has consumed much energy and probably represents a truce rather than an equilibrium, with the potential for breaking down under the sort of pressure that would arise if general practice were expected to increase its work-load still further without the provision of the resources to enable it to do so.

This book seeks to name the core values of practitioners and the core values of practices, in the belief that each is appropriate in its appropriate context. Understanding and honouring both sets of values should help all who work in general practice to make sense of and resolve the confusion, conflicts and unease currently experienced. Practitioner and practice values must also be understood and valued by NHS managers if general practice is to play its part in the 'strategic shift' to a primary health care led NHS.

Summary of values

In describing core general practice, we can distinguish between practitioners, who work in one-to-one relationships with patients responding to their concerns, and the practice, an organization with wider concerns, particularly for improving the health of its registered population of patients with the available resources. Once this distinction has been made, it is clear that there are important differences in underlying core values. Practitioner and practice values are summarized in Table 1.1 and are explored in the body of this report.

Table 1.1   A summary of practitioner and practice values

Practitioner values	Practice values
The patient: Recognizing patients as whole people, and acceptance of any problem they choose to bring	The population: Recognizing the registered practice population as a whole and accepting responsibility for its health and health care
• broad remit	• broader remit, including health
• relationship with whole person, whether or not problems correspond to biomedical diagnoses	• responsibility to the population of registered patients, whether or not they consult
• unconditional advocate of individual patients	• fair distribution of resources
• responsibility for co-ordination of individual's care	• managing the coherence of connections

Table 1.1 *continued*

Practitioner values	Practice values
The practitioner: Maintaining the quality of the practitioner	*The practice: Maintaining the quality of the organization*

• technical competence
  – qualification and training
  – professional accountability
  – professional audit
  – relationship with specialists
  – continuing education
  – managing time
	• organizational competence
	  – systems and communication
	  – contractual responsibility
	  – audit (interprofessional)
	  – connections with the system
	  – developmental capacity (adaptive)
	  – managing resource use

• physical wellbeing	• buildings, equipment, appropriate work-load
• emotional wellbeing	• safe, supportive environment
• spiritual wellbeing	• vision/measures of success
The intent: Action in the best interests of the individual patient	*The intent: Action in the best interests of the registered practice population*
• using available resources to improve wellbeing of individual patients	• using available resources to maximize health gain for the population – equity

• recognizing and overriding conflict of interest between patient and practitioner
  – honesty
  – avoiding exploitation
	• recognizing and overriding conflict of interest between the practice population and the practice itself
	  – putting interests of patients before practice finances

Table 1.1 *continued*

Practitioner values	Practice values
• recognizing and addressing conflict of interest between patient and other individuals, including family – confidentiality – supporting patient in resolving conflicts	• recognizing and addressing conflict of interest between the whole population and individuals – tailoring care and services to need rather than demand
• accountability to patient – partnership, informed consent	• accountability to users/representatives
• accountability to profession	• accountability to health commissions
• limited proactive role – exploring unexpressed health needs sensitively	• extended proactive role – systematic health needs assessment
• limited prevention and health promotion in the interests of the individual	• systematic prevention and health promotion, when justified by risk–benefit and cost–benefit
The means: The consultation	*The means: Providing, commissioning and alliances*
• personal care	• division of labour, teamwork
• continuity of care	• care by the most appropriately skilled
• availability of individual practitioners	• access by whole practice population
• advocacy for individuals	• advocacy for population, rationing
• effectiveness as a significant factor	• effectiveness as a key factor
• efficiency as a by-product of good practice	• efficiency as driving force

Table 1.1 *continued*

Practitioner values	Practice values
• clinical records	• information systems, call and recall
• appropriate referral	• commissioning appropriate secondary care
• mutual trust	• 'power over'
• toleration of uncertainty	• wider alliances for health promotion
• intimacy and emotional awareness	• intersectoral (multiagency) working
• empowerment	• political action

Conflicts of values

The values described here by the term practitioner are broadly those of the family doctor, whereas the values described by the term practice are broadly those of the new public health. In many situations, the two sets of values support each other in constructive tension. However, the wants of individuals are not compatible invariably with their needs as assessed by another or with the needs of a population. In these situations, the two sets of values are in conflict.

This may be apparent whenever services are rationed. If a practitioner spends time working to improve the population health, that time is not available for individual patients. The conflict is apparent most obviously if a practitioner (whose value system requires her to represent the interest of her *individual* patient) is involved with the practice task of the allocation of funds for secondary care among the *population* of patients (as may occur, for example, in fundholding practices).

Even when rationing is not the issue, there is a balance to be achieved between continuity of care (a practitioner value) and care by a multiprofessional team (a practice value). Where this balance has been distorted by the requirements of finance and short-term 'efficiency', the values of practitioner and practice will be at odds.

Many practitioners are at present trying to honour both sets of values simultaneously, without always acknowledging the area of conflict. Practitioners may feel more comfortable and work more effectively if they choose to identify with *either* the practitioner *or* the practice roles and values.

The core general practitioner: the doctor, the patient and the illness

2

This chapter considers the core values of the practitioner, while Chapter 3 considers the core values of the practice and Chapter 4 the ways in which these sets of values can support each other most productively.

Most one-to-one consultations in general practice are with doctors, so this chapter begins by looking at the context in which the general practitioner role developed. It then builds up a model of the practitioner. The Capital Conferences named biomedical and biographical aspects of the practitioner and described features that lie outside these aspects and seem to fall into two separate groups, described as the aspects of 'carer' and 'healer'. The chapter closes by bringing these aspects together in a model of the practitioner and naming its underlying values.

The context of development

In 1948, general practitioners chose a semi-detached relationship with the NHS. The need to negotiate an independent contractor status arose, at least in part, from the perception of many GPs that a salaried service would lead to a loss of clinical freedom. The GP was seen frequently as the 'poor relation' of the hospital consultant, reflecting the historical relationship of apothecary and physician. A coalition of interests enshrined the role of the GP as gatekeeper to specialist care and thus prepared the ground for GPs, at a later date, to become involved in the rationing of secondary care.

During the early years, there was widespread disillusionment among GPs about 'this nationalized health service', resulting in substantial emigration. If generalists were thought to be providing merely a cheap and second-rate version of specialist care, did they have any role when payment at the point of delivery of health care had been abolished?

During the 1950s and 1960s, British general practice developed a vision of what it might mean to be a clinical generalist within a national health service and how this role could be developed. The vision was pursued, using professional mechanisms, by the formation of the Royal College of General Practitioners (RCGP), its development of membership by examination and the pioneering of vocational training. The same vision was accepted by the General Medical Services Committee of the British Medical Association (GMSC), and the 1966 Charter for general practice resulted in public spending on general practice buildings, staff and equipment.

Perhaps the most familiar statements of essential values in general practice at that time first appeared in 1972 in *The future general practitioner. Learning and teaching*[5] and then in the European Leeuwenhorst Working Party statement of 1977[6]:

> 'The General Practitioner is a licensed medical graduate who gives personal, primary and continuing care to individuals, families and a practice population, irrespective of age, sex and illness. It is the synthesis of these functions which is unique'.

Here the general practitioner is described as providing care for 'individuals, families and populations' (Figure 1). When there are conflicts of interest within families, practitioners may feel able to act in the best interests of whichever family member

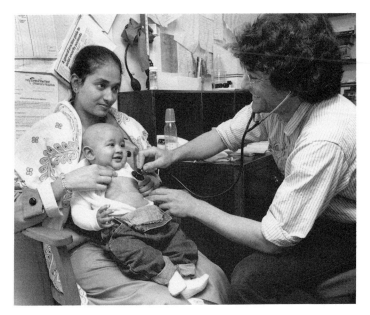

Figure 1

is consulting at that moment. Patients will, however, often feel most comfortable if each has their own confidential advocate. This can occur within a practice of more than one doctor without any departure from practitioner values. The inclusion of 'care to the practice population' in the Leeuwenhorst statement acknowledges that the development of some of what are here described as practice values was already well established by 1977.

The biomedical aspect

Doctors have, during the last century, been trained principally in the 'biomedical' model, in which the application of the scientific method to medical care has proved to be immensely powerful in the understanding, prevention and treatment of *diseases*. The biomedical approach provides a shared base of knowledge that allows the physician to make statistical predictions of the prognosis of the patient's disease and to make objectively justifiable diagnostic and therapeutic decisions. The strength of the biomedical physician lies in an ability to 'get it right' at an intellectual level.

The biomedical approach is not peculiar to doctors and nurses, being employed by many of the professions supplementary to medicine, such as physiotherapy and dietetics. When asked to explain why a particular intervention is used, a biomedical practitioner will explain his or her approach in terms of ideas, models, techniques and evidence – that is to say, the approach relies on the *mind* of the practitioner (by contrast with the emotions, body or spirit). In this respect, it has much in common with a range of techniques that may be considered to lie on the periphery of the biomedical approach, ranging from cognitive therapy, through relaxation and visualization, to hypnotic suggestion. It has some similarities with a range of 'complementary' or 'alternative' therapies (such as osteopathy, chiropractic, acupuncture and homeopathy), each of which has its own knowledge-base.

The core values of all biomedical practitioners include technical competence and action in the perceived best interests of the individual patient. These are reflected in the medical profession's self-regulatory concern with standards of training and qualification and in the ethical areas of confidentiality, informed consent and forbidding exploitation of the relationship, particularly for financial, emotional or sexual gain.

Biomedical physician as clinical generalist

Two factors, in particular, limit the applicability of this bio-medical approach to *all* situations in which people feel ill and distressed.

- Much of the illness that patients bring to professionals is not directly related to disease states that are amenable to biomedical intervention.

- Biomedical investigations and treatments can be hazard-ous, as well as expensive and time-consuming.

It is, therefore, important to limit the use of the biomedical approach to situations in which its benefits outweigh its risks and warrant its costs. One factor that has helped its appropriate application has been the development of both clinical gener-alists and specialists, each of whom works in a way that is appropriate to the differing disease prevalences in the popu-lations in which they practise. Iona Heath has described the general practitioner as the 'guardian of the interface between illness and disease'[7].

The knowledge- and skills-base of biomedical science has, in this century, become so extensive that there is a need for specialists. There are, in principle, two ways in which patients can relate to a range of biomedical specialists. They can, as is common in the USA, decide themselves which specialty is likely to be appropriate to their illness and rely on the specialist to manage within his own specialty and/or suggest consulting a different specialist. Alternatively, they can, as is usual in the UK, consult a generalist who is able to manage common problems and who knows when it is appropriate to seek referral and to which specialist. A particular strength of this latter approach derives from the experience that many patients bring problems from more than one specialty. These problems are connected, at the very least, by occurring in the same person. This requires that the generalist have a broad remit, to make appropriate use of referral to secondary care and thus to take responsibility for co-ordination of care. As the first port of call for most health problems, it also requires availability of access to the generalist for all patients.

Generalists have the role of reducing risk to the patient that may arise either from treatable disease, on the one hand, or from medical intervention, on the other. In populations with a low prevalence of treatable disease (such as the unselected patients of a general practice), this requires generalists to accept some diagnostic uncertainty in order to protect their patients from the hazards of medical intervention. Where the patient's condition indicates that there is a significant risk of harm to the patient, a generalist will pursue diagnostic certainty by performing investigations and sometimes by referring the patient to a specialist. She may also pursue diagnostic certainty if that is what the patient wishes or needs for reassurance. Marshall Marinker has described this role as 'to accept uncertainty, to explore probability and to marginalise danger'[8].

An essential attribute of the generalist is to be able to tolerate uncertainty and to enable the patient to do the same. Living with uncertainty requires mutual trust and a willingness to re-evaluate the situation as it develops over time. Continuity of care facilitates this generalist role, both because it provides the framework for re-evaluation and because it gives rise to a personal relationship in which mutual trust can begin to develop.

Specialists have the role of eliminating uncertainty, as is appropriate for the populations they are dealing with – those selected by generalists to include a high prevalence of disease. By performing a series of investigations to 'exclude' disease, they are able to say authoritatively whether the patient has a disease described within their specialty and, if so, to name it. They accept the risks and costs of investigation, as necessary, to fulfil their role – 'to reduce uncertainty, to explore possibility and to marginalise error'.

One of the consequences of specialists dealing directly with patients who refer themselves, rather than with those selected by generalists, is that they may apply their uncertainty-reducing strategies and investigate (and treat) more extensively than would a generalist. There are likely to be fewer missed diagnoses but a higher level of iatrogenic illness, more referrals between specialists and a more costly service[9]. There will be differing views as to which is more appropriate – a specialist or a generalist service in primary care.

> The values of the clinical generalist thus include, in addition to those of all biomedical practitioners, accepting any problem brought by the patient that might be amenable to biomedical intervention (broad biomedical remit), availability, *mutual* trust, continuity of care, responsibility for co-ordination of care of the individual patient and the ability to tolerate uncertainty.

Problems for the clinical generalist

Toleration of uncertainty

Tolerating uncertainty is demanding and requires training, experience, mutual trust between practitioner and patient, and supportive specialist colleagues. Above all, it requires appropriate self-confidence, an ability to reflect on the complexities of the presenting situation and a sense of balance on the tight-rope of each consultation. It is an aspect of the consultation in which the locus of control must be managed carefully – uncertainty may be inappropriately held by the practitioner or imposed on the patient, instead of being shared appropriately.

In order to tolerate uncertainty within the consultation, the GP is likely to have a psychological need for some certainty in the structures in which consultations are embedded. General practitioners coping with the uncertainties induced by the NHS reforms are unlikely to feel able to tolerate such high levels of uncertainty as previously.

Inappropriate toleration of uncertainty

Just as the generalist may over-investigate, over-refer and over-treat, so also may she under-investigate, under-refer and under-treat. Such errors of omission are much more visible than are errors of commission. When the errors are shared with peers or patients through informal discussions or audit, specific action may be taken to prevent their re-occurrence. When the errors are revealed by complaints or litigation, it is likely to result in a reduced ability to tolerate uncertainty and the practice of 'defensive medicine'.

Effectiveness

If a practitioner were to make use only of the biomedical approach, it might be expected that she would employ only therapeutic interventions of proven effectiveness – that is to say, those which have been demonstrated in randomized controlled trials to have greater success than a placebo. This approach is most easily sustained by the specialist, who may legitimately terminate a professional relationship if he or she feels that the biomedical approach within the specialty has nothing further to offer that patient. For all practitioners, but particularly for the generalist in a continuing relationship with a patient, there are good reasons for using interventions not known to be effective, as described below. However, there are also bad reasons, one of which is an unquestioning attitude encouraged by an undergraduate medical education that relies on the acceptance of received wisdom in clinical practice, leaving the doctor susceptible to influence by the pharmaceutical industry. Another is the use of a prescription as a substitute for more appropriate action (such as listening, explaining or examining), particularly to shorten a consultation.

A good reason for using interventions of unknown or questionable effectiveness is the desire to care for the patient (described as the 'carer' aspect of the practitioner), which may manifest as 'doing something'. A hand on the patient's forehead is not 'effective' treatment for vomiting, in the sense that this intervention has not been subjected to a randomized controlled trial, but it frequently makes the patient feel more comfortable. Indeed, the feeling of being cared for (and about), and the improved sense of comfort, may reduce the vomiting itself. The practitioner may use a prescription in the same way, as a way of caring.

An overlapping but separate reason is the ambiguous position of the placebo response in the understanding of effectiveness. Where there is no treatment of known effectiveness, clinical trials compare treatment with placebo, yet it is known that the rate of response to placebo for a very wide range of symptoms is of the order of 15–30%[10]. Given this knowledge, it would actually be irrational, even within the biomedical model, *not* to use therapeutic interventions of doubtful effectiveness in appropriate situations, provided that the placebo effectiveness outweighs the risks and warrants the costs. Working consciously with this knowledge is an important contemporary challenge within the biomedical approach. The problem for clinical generalists working in this way is that biomedical treatments are usually associated with significant risks and costs. It could be argued that generalists, in order to maximize their caring and placebo effectiveness, need to have available treatments of negligible risk, low cost and unproven (but believable) effectiveness.

> For these reasons, the values of the clinical generalist include the provision of effective care, but effectiveness, narrowly defined, is not the sole criterion for deciding whether or not to use a particular treatment.

The biographical aspect

Working as clinical generalists, general practitioners became aware of the limited appropriateness of the biomedical model to the ill-defined and complex problems that were brought to them every day. They developed a theoretical framework to use this lack of definition in a positive way, rather than seeing it as an impediment to good biomedical practice. This framework was described and developed in a number of publications, including *The future general practitioner*[5] and *The doctor, his patient and the illness*, by Michael Balint[11]. Balint observed that patients presented frequently, not with disease states, formulated and ready to be processed within the biomedical model, but with illness, dis-ease and 'messy' problems that required clarification, interpretation and negotiation as to their meaning and significance. Balint pointed out that an experienced general practitioner accepts whatever complaints or symptoms the patient brings and works with the patient, for example by paraphrasing and reflecting back, to enable her to make sense of the problems and to take appropriate action. This approach, focusing on the patient's biography, respects the uniqueness and continuity of a patient's life and the importance of the patient's life story[12].

The term 'biographical' refers here to practitioners' use of the biographical approach. In order to bring to the surface the life experience, emotions and intuitions of their patients, they will need to be aware of their own life experience, emotions and intuitions, accepting the intimacy of each encounter, within the context of the consultation (Figure 2). The intimacy

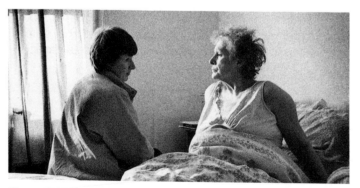

Figure 2

of this way of working is what binds many GPs to their work but it is not easy to communicate to somebody who has not experienced it (Figure 3). It cannot be appreciated without sensitive observation and recording of anecdote, within the context of a wider view. It is described by Huygen in *Family medicine, the medical life histories of families*[13] and illustrated by John Berger and Jean Mohr in *A fortunate man, the story of a country doctor*[14] and by David Widgery in *Some lives!*[15].

More generally, the biographical approach is one that makes use of the emotions of the practitioner. It is used extensively by psychotherapists and also by some complementary practitioners, social workers and counsellors.

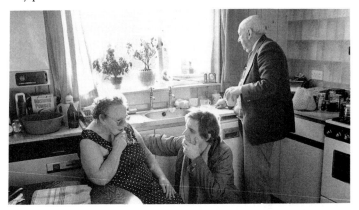

Figure 3

The values of the biographical practitioner will include the primacy of the consultation; acceptance of the whole person and any problems he or she may choose to bring, even where these do not fit within the biomedical model; intimacy and emotional awareness; shared understanding of the problem; consensus regarding management; and the continuity of care that makes it possible to put these values into practice.

Problems for the biographical practitioner

Inappropriate application

The general practitioner tries to hold in balance the biographical and biomedical aspects of care. Many consultations require a stepping to and fro between these aspects, and there is a constant risk of employing the inappropriate one. If a GP fails to maintain the balance and systematically neglects the biomedical role, it is dangerous for patients and undermines the expectations on which the relationship is based.

Training and support

To work within the biographical aspects requires interaction at an emotional level with large numbers of patients. Psychotherapists working in this way, for example, are aware of the need not only for training in the techniques used, but also for personal therapy and supervision. This gives the therapist insight and support in conducting the therapeutic session and, in particular, in issues relating to boundaries, transference and counter-transference. Many GPs have received relatively little training for this role and are, perhaps in consequence, often not open to personal therapy or supervision.

Being valued by self and others

The core values of practitioners are expressed unobserved in the privacy of the consultation, which means that it is very important for practitioners to be able to value themselves and to be valued by their patients. This sense of being valued by equals differs from and complements the hierarchical nature of value that is found within the biomedical tradition, for example by specialist colleagues who understand and appreciate the role of the generalist practitioner, rather than viewing her as one with an inferior knowledge of their specialty.

While biographical practitioners value the work they do using the approach, there are major problems in its application within time-limited services. Although it can lead to rapid diagnostic and therapeutic insights, most practitioners working in this way find that it adds to the length of consultations. A biographical practitioner may decide not to follow directions in the consultation that she suspects would be useful, solely because of lack of time. This sense of having to provide a safe but second-best service leads to a loss of self-valuation. Whereas it has been possible, in the past, for some practitioners to compensate for the variable time pressures by offering 'a long appointment next week', the increase in non-consultation work-load[16] and the increased numbers of patients seen by doctors in clinics[17] now makes this option less possible.

The biographical approach requires a partnership between practitioner and patient. Some specialists, managers and even GPs have a past experience of predominantly unequal relationships between practitioners and patients that makes it difficult for them to understand and appreciate this approach.

The caring aspect

A human response to the illness and distress of others that is recognized generally is to care for them – to provide physical and emotional support. At times, this may involve taking action, 'doing something', whereas at others, it may involve simply being there, continuing to accept the patient unconditionally, without judgement. Most fundamentally, it involves caring *about* another, feeling with them.

Most caring is provided by family and friends. Within the primary health care team, the member with the most important caring role is the district nurse. In the practice itself, GPs and practice nurses make a small but often crucial contribution. Empathy in consultation, a practical procedure performed sensitively or an unrequested home visit in times of distress are felt by most patients to be important contributions to care (Figure 4). People want to be recognized for their

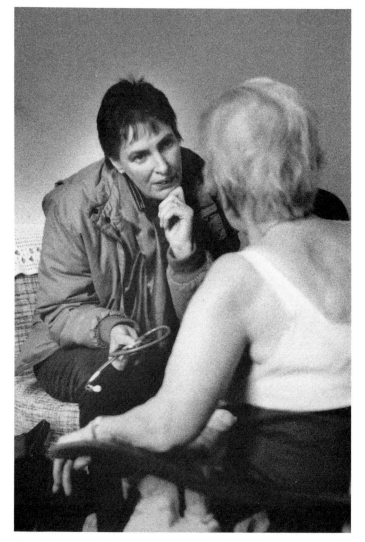

Figure 4

intrinsic value as individuals and will be disappointed or even repelled by a health worker if this recognition is lacking.

> The core value of the carer is that of putting the needs of the patient first; in order to achieve this, the carer needs to take care of her own wellbeing, particularly at the physical and emotional level – which is sometimes described as 'self-gardening'[18].

Problems for the carer

Paternalism and the creation of dependence

Where caring involves acting for patients over a period of time, there is a risk that patients may inappropriately let go of responsibility for themselves, becoming dependent and disempowered. This undermines not only the patients' autonomy but also their self-healing potential.

In a parallel development, the practitioner may adopt a paternalistic approach, inappropriately taking 'power over', rather than empowering the patient.

Exhaustion

Caring may involve giving physical or emotional energy. If this continues over time without rest and rebuilding the energy by self-gardening, the carer will become exhausted.

The healing aspect

Before the development of the biomedical approach, people turned in times of illness to 'medicine men' (or women), the traditional healers, whose way of working includes using that aspect of themselves that is referred to as 'the spirit'.

Some readers may feel that the practitioner can be described adequately by the three aspects (caring, biomedical and biographical) described already. Others[19] may feel that as well as using their bodies, minds and emotions in these aspects, there are occasions when their spirits may be employed for the purposes of healing. Perhaps the clearest way of describing this approach is at the level of meaning.

In the biomedical aspect, the meaning of symptoms is provided in terms of verifiable causes, for example physical traumas, infective agents, genetic abnormalities, environmental pollutants and social conditions. In the biographical aspect, the meaning of symptoms is provided by accepting the legitimacy of the past life experience of the individual patient. In the practitioner's caring aspect, the meaning is provided by her actions at that moment, by the present reality of physical and emotional security within an ongoing relationship. However, these aspects of meaning provide only very partial answers to the frequent questions 'Why me?' and 'Why now?'. By turning to another in search of meanings that illuminate the purpose of life and the steps on a path through it, a patient is seeking out a healer.

A healer recognizes the individuality and wholeness of her patients, acting as a witness to their life, illness and death and thus enabling each to appreciate their own special nature, while connecting with the universal experience of what it is to be human. Healers enable their patients to connect with their own belief system and thus with positive states, such as awareness of the self as part of the universe, being in the present, understanding the inevitability of change and accepting adversity as learning. People seek out as healers others who have asked themselves similar questions about meaning and who appear to be at peace with themselves.

This is an aspect that is, perhaps, not in great demand in our society, and to the extent that it is supplied, its practitioners are likely to be spiritual and religious leaders. However, patients sometimes seem to want their practitioner to work in this way at the particular times in their lives, such as birth, death and bereavement, when they are most closely in touch with their own self and the meaning of their own lives.

> The core values of the healer include a keen awareness of the connections between people and between people and the universe; a desire to enable patients to take as much responsibility for self-healing as they can handle on that occasion; and caring for the integrity and wellbeing of the healer him- or herself, particularly at the spiritual level.

The practitioner's core values

The practitioner

The practitioner has the potential to synthesize the four aspects (biomedical, biographical, caring and healing) in working with the body, mind, emotions and spirit of a whole patient. This can be represented diagrammatically as in Figure 5.

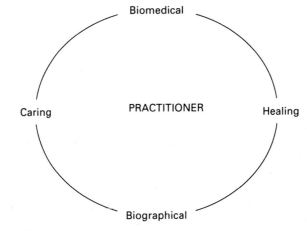

Figure 5

Each aspect of this model has its own different associated skills and values. At different times, the practitioner needs to work in different aspects, and there is considerable skill in deciding which aspect to use when. This is particularly the case when there is some conflict between the values underlying the different aspects.

This model illustrates the potential for the practitioner and the consultation. The practitioner may be working with any combination of the four aspects of the core. Most GPs will be likely to employ the biomedical approach extensively, as this is a major element in training, and the healing aspect rather little. In each consultation, the GP is likely to be moving to and fro between the aspects – now pursuing a diagnosis (biomedical), now exploring anxieties (biographical), now performing a physical examination (biomedical), now providing practical help (caring) and now 'being there' as a witness to the life of the individual patient (healing). The biomedical aspect is fundamental to the expectations of both doctor and patient in general practice in our society – doctors are registered on the basis of this aspect of their practice and this is the unique aspect that patients can obtain from nobody else[20].

Anthony Rooley in *Performance – Revealing the Orpheus Within*, describes three 'principles' in performance described in the early sixteenth century, whether this be the performance of music or the experience of life, which may perhaps be applied to the consultation. The first principle, decoro, refers to those aspects of performance that are based in appropriate technique and can be developed by teaching and practice. The dominant part of the biomedical approach lies within this principle, and it is also employed in the biographical and caring approaches. The second, balancing principle, sprezzatura, refers to a bold, intuitive, excitement in the moment that is prepared to embrace the unknown. At times needed in the biomedical approach, this is an essential aspect of the caring and biographical approaches. Rooley describes a third, fundamental, principle, grazia, which belongs to no one, will not manifest itself on request but, when present, is instantly recognized. This may be what is needed for healing.

This model of the four aspects also represents, in most consultations, an ideal rather than a reality, and there is a danger in describing an ideal in case it becomes the enemy of the 'good enough'[21]. However, with this proviso, it may prove useful, not least in explaining the potential richness of the consultation.

The model has been derived from the experience of general practitioners but is not unique to them. Other health and social care workers have developed aspects of the caring, healing, biomedical and biographical approaches more fully than have general practitioners. Each such group of workers will find a different balance of, and different ways of working within, the four aspects; for example, the medical specialist will place more emphasis on the biomedical, the psychotherapist more on the biographical and the district nurse more on the caring aspect.

Before summarizing the values of the practitioner, it should be reiterated that the term 'practitioner' is used in this book to include not only GPs, but also all those who work in general practice and have a one-to-one relationship with patients. Doctors, nurses and counsellors are all likely to identify broadly with practitioner values in their individual relationships with patients.

Receptionists are not usually described as practitioners, and their one-to-one relationships with patients are conducted in public. However, they may take on any of the aspects of the practitioner at some times. Consider, for example, the response of an experienced receptionist to the arrival of a patient with chest pain and their distressed spouse. A receptionist balancing one patient's request for attention by the doctor with the efficient running of the practice as a whole is balancing practitioner and practice values.

The values

Having considered separately the core values of the biomedical, biographical, caring and healing aspects, it is possible to bring them together and find important differences, yet to be aware that they are interdependent and need to be held in balance with each other. Practitioners struggle to manage this tension creatively. The values are summarized in Table 2.1, divided for the sake of clarity into values relating to the patient, the practitioner, the practitioner's intent and the means (or way of working).

Table 2.1   A summary of practitioner values

The patient: Recognizing patients as whole people, and acceptance of any problem they choose to bring
- broad remit
- relationship with whole person, whether or not problems correspond to biomedical diagnoses
- unconditional advocate of individual patients
- responsibility for co-ordination of individual's care

The practitioner: Maintaining the quality of the practitioner
- technical competence
  - qualification and training
  - professional accountability
  - professional audit
  - relationship with specialists
  - continuing education
  - managing time
- physical wellbeing
- emotional wellbeing
- spiritual wellbeing

The intent: Action in the best interests of the individual patient
- using available resources to improve wellbeing of individual patients

Table 2.1 *continued*

- recognizing and overriding conflict of interest between patient and practitioner
  - honesty
  - avoiding exploitation

- recognizing and overriding conflict of interest between the patient and other individuals, including family
  - confidentiality
  - supporting patients in resolving problems

- accountability to patient
  - partnership, informed consent

- accountability to profession
- limited proactive role
  - exploring unexpressed health needs sensitively

- limited prevention and health promotion in the interests of the individual

The means: The consultation
- personal care
- continuity of care
- availability of individual practitioners
- advocacy for individuals
- effectiveness as a significant factor
- efficiency as a by-product of good practice
- clinical records
- appropriate referral
- mutual trust, empathy
- toleration of uncertainty
- intimacy and emotional awareness
- empowerment

Core general practice: the practice, its population and their health

Chapter 2 examined the values of the practitioner; Chapter 3 examines the values of the practice. It begins by looking at the factors that have influenced the development of the general practice. It then describes three roles for the practice: to influence health, to deal with populations and to function as an organization. It concludes by examining the values that are required to fill these roles, analysing the practice using a model similar to that developed for the practitioner.

The role of the practitioner is encompassed by the idea of the family doctor and the role of the practice in the new public health. Just as the phrase 'The doctor, his patient and the illness' is used to illuminate the role of the practitioner, so the role of the practice can be illuminated by the phrase 'The practice, its population and their health'[22]. These are two distinct roles that potentially conflict. Not only are the roles different, but so also is the audience to which they are directed; while the former is addressed to practitioners, the latter is addressed to the commissioners of primary health care.

The context of development

The transition from individual practitioner to organization can be broadly analysed as two stages. In the first stage (up to the late 1980s), it was driven from within the medical profession and affected only a proportion of practices. In the second (from 1990), it affected all practices and was driven by a change in the role of the state in general and public sector providers in particular.

Development of general practice by general practitioners

Collaboration between GPs, as with some apothecaries before them, started with very small partnerships, which developed after the Second World War into larger groups. This enabled GPs to make more 'efficient' use of their time (eg sharing night duties) and resources (eg premises and receptionists). The development of multiprofessional groups that followed was a response both to the increase in demand from patients and to the increased number and range of interventions that biomedical and social science had made possible, particularly in prevention, health education and counselling. This resulted in the health centre movement and ultimately in the 1966 Charter for family doctors[23].

Growing numbers of GPs, supported by the Royal College of General Practitioners[24], were aware of the social and economic causes of ill health and pioneered the population view of their practice lists, developing strategies for prevention and the promotion of health in general practice. However, by the end of the 1980s, the further development of general practice appeared to be slow and uncertain. Practices keen to develop a full range of services were held back by the limits on the numbers of staff they were assisted to employ. They were able to employ the necessary staff only where a Family

Practitioner Committee was prepared to use 'flexibility' in its interpretation of the Statement of Fees and Allowances (Red Book) provisions for the payment of ancillary staff, where a health authority was unusually imaginative in its attachment of staff, where funding was available from outside the NHS (eg charities, Healthy City projects or Regional Arts) or where the doctors chose to take a lower rate of pay than they would expect in otherwise comparable practices.

General practices, like other small organizations in which control is held by a small group with a long-term commitment, developed a traditional management style. However, practices often seemed to be held back by this central role of the GP within the organization[25]. The doctor's position as the employer leads to an imbalance of power that makes it difficult to take on the role of team member, and the role of team leader may also be compromised. GP negotiators had insisted on retaining the independent contractor status and on contracting as individuals rather than as organizations. Contracting as an individual to provide a population approach to health as well as health care requires practitioners to identify with the values that are appropriate to the practice (Figure 6).

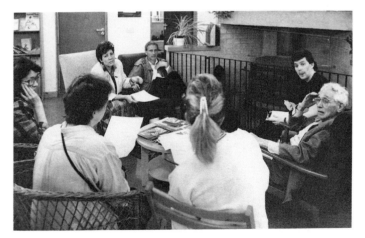

Figure 6

Some practices in the late 1980s were showing no signs of taking on the population and health perspectives espoused by the leaders of the profession, or even of developing teamwork within their organization. This was the state of general practice when its foundations were rocked by the impact of a new set of priorities sweeping the whole of the public sector.

Development of general practice and the 'new public management'

The public sector in the UK has been subjected to far-reaching management reforms since 1979, driven by the desire of government to generate 'good management' in the public sector and variously described as the 'financial management initiative' (FMI), 'next steps' or the 'new public management'. The reforms are based on the assumptions that:

- 'bad management' existed in public sector service units before the reforms

- the private sector has 'good management' in place

- the success of management in the private sector is due to the fact that it has FMI-type management structures and behaviour.

The key features of FMI, as described by Laughlin and Broadbent[26] are:

1 financial devolution to units directly offering services

2 explicit standards and measures of performance for these units

3 clear relationships between inputs, outputs and performance measures for the units

4 increased accountability requirements from these units

5 stress on private sector styles of management

6 stress on competition and contracting between units

7 stress on efficiency and parsimony in resource usage.

Implicit in this approach is the decentralized model of divisionalization, in which budgetary control is delegated to the divisions, which are deemed to be better attuned to their local environment and which can, therefore, make 'better' decisions. This apparent freedom is accompanied by constraints about what the devolved unit should be doing. It is this pattern of apparent freedom, yet increased measurable control, that is at the heart of FMI.

The implications of this devolution of responsibility are felt most keenly in the arena of resource allocation (rationing). The FMI model retains control of overall levels of expenditure but devolves responsibility for resource allocation to a more local level. This produces a lack of clarity, and thus lack of public accountability, about whether the under-provision of a particular service is due to a central decision about overall levels of funding or to local variations in priorities, efficiencies, health needs and ease of delivering services.

In the NHS, most but not all of these elements of the FMI were put in place by the National Health Service and Community Care Act (1990) and the 1990 GP contract. The stress on competition and contracting (feature 6) requires the operation of a market. The 'internal market' created by the reforms, which provided a mechanism for financial devolution (feature 1) to take place, is not, however, a free market in the economic sense. While a true free market would rely on market processes to express values, the internal market has to define quantifiable output measures and performance measures (feature 2) as a proxy for value. These proxies for value are then used for decision-making (feature 3) and to provide accountability (feature 4).

An example of a performance measure used in secondary care is the 'finished consultant episode'. If measures as crude as the 'consultation episode' were to be introduced into general practice, it is difficult to imagine that they could be shown to correlate other than negatively with any measure of the value of the consultations, as assessed by patients or doctors.

Output and performance measures for contract monitoring (features 2 and 3) are at present based on readily available data (eg immunization and cervical cytology targets and drug costs), which reflect only a small part of the activity of practitioners. These proxies for value are not measuring aspects of the work of general practitioners that are considered to be at the core of their role, although, as we shall see, they do measure aspects of the work of the practice. This gives a strong message that practitioners and their consultations are not a valued part of the practice in which they work and leads to a transfer of resources and time away from individual patient care.

It is possible to try to assess the quality of the work of the practitioner using methods such as those used for the assessment of teaching practices and assessment of the quality of the consultation (eg The Leicester Assessment Package[27]). These methods are used most appropriately in the context of professional development and self-regulation. Their use for contract monitoring could provide more appropriate measures of practitioner performance than those currently in use but might require greater trust between practitioners and health commissions than would be appropriate.

The limits to economic reason

The FMI places 'economic reason' at the core of health care provision, and it is not self-evident that this is appropriate. Although economic reason may appear to be neutral, it carries its own values, particularly the value that it is possible to put a price on everything of importance. The models employed in economic science, particularly those at the heart of the free market model, assume a sphere of activity, 'the economy', in which people take on simple roles (eg producer or consumer) and behave 'rationally' within the roles, that is to say, use 'economic reason'. However, many spheres of our lives are predominantly influenced by factors (eg relationships, beliefs and ethics) other than economic 'rationality'. For example, while a practitioner functions within the economy (she is remunerated for her work and responds to financial 'carrots' as well as contractual 'sticks'), she has also 'been involved in the service she has provided in a manner that can neither be *produced* at will, nor bought, learned or codified. She has shown an interest in the other person as a human being and not just in their money; she has established a relationship with the other that cannot be expressed in terms of pre-defined technical procedure or computer program'[28]. That is to say, her core values are not determined by economic reason alone.

Economic reason requires products that are measurable, so that they can be assigned a price and put out to contract. This approach is not incompatible fundamentally with the biomedical aspects of the practitioner's role, as the rationale for such measurements arises from the same positivist tradition. It is, however, incompatible with the biographical and healing aspects of the practitioner, which see the patient as a self-healing organism and health as a process, rather than a product.

Laughlin and Broadbent suggest that in health care and education, as in the church, the core values and practice are felt to be sacred, while the peripheral activities are felt to be secular or profane. Where economic reason enters core activities, it may be perceived as a secularization process that has the potential for destroying the sacred core.

Although economic reason is at times incompatible with the core values of the practitioner, there is no such incompatibility with the core values of the practice. The practice is an organization that must satisfy its commissioners or fail financially, so must have values that are congruent with the health commission. This will include the acceptance of economic reason, unless it can persuade the commission to 'buy into' the values of the practitioner.

Levels of resources

The apparent neutrality of economic reason can be used to effect change in the priorities and core values of an organization. The 1990 contract funded the responsibility of the practice for the health of the population by withdrawing funding from practitioner care[29], and thereby effected a shift in values within the practice.

Another resource-led development that has tended to reinforce practice values has been the control of drug costs by indicative prescribing amounts. Limiting the budget for drugs has the desirable effect of encouraging practice formularies, generic prescribing and rational prescribing. Once this step has been taken, the only ways of further reducing costs are to stop prescribing drugs that the patient can buy over the counter and to prescribe cheaper treatment that is known to be less effective. As the indicative prescribing amounts were introduced on the basis of historical prescribing costs, some practitioners found that limited resources forced the practitioner to adopt practice values when making prescribing decisions, by putting population needs above the wellbeing of individual patients.

In examining the difference between practitioner (doctor, patient and illness) and practice (practice, population and health) we shall consider first the change from 'the illness' to 'their health'.

From 'the illness' to 'their health'

The health of a population can be improved by treating illness, preventing disease and promoting health. Treatment and prevention are compatible with the biomedical model in which 'health' is residual once disease has been eliminated. Health promotion is derived from a different view of health as a dynamic equilibrium of wellbeing, capable of encompassing every aspect of life, from the environment to communities, from employment to personal sense of worth and direction (Figure 7).

Treatment of illness, according to the pure biomedical model, requires that the patient's illness should fit the labelling criteria of one of the available diseases. Conditions that do not meet this criterion are accepted only so that biomedical diagnoses can be 'excluded'. Consultations should result in a positive diagnosis or the 'exclusion' of a condition of biomedical importance; otherwise, they risk the description of 'unnecessary'. The biographical practitioner goes a long way towards accepting whatever the patient chooses to bring, but even here, the patient will often feel the need to bring a physical symptom as a 'passport' to the consultation.

Prevention of disease may be divided into primary prevention (reducing risk of developing disease, eg immunization and dietary/smoking/exercise advice), secondary prevention (early diagnosis and treatment of disease, eg cervical smears, mammography and the treatment of hypertension) and tertiary prevention (preventing disability and the deterioration of existing disease). Tertiary, secondary and even primary prevention lie within the personal sphere and the biomedical model. On an individual rather than a population level, prevention has been an important part of the consultations of the practitioner. The relationships and contacts arising from patients' felt needs can be used to involve them in activities that prevent disease and are understood to be clearly in their own interest.

Promotion of health looks beyond one individual and one disease. It empowers individuals or groups to develop their own health as they see it, to look to wider causes of illness and distress, taking action to address these issues (eg income support, unemployment, housing, health and safety at work, pollution, availability of healthy foods, cigarette advertising, access to leisure facilities and road safety issues). Promotion of health is likely to require collaborative, intersectoral and political actions. There are examples of general practices that have taken this approach to their population's health[30], but

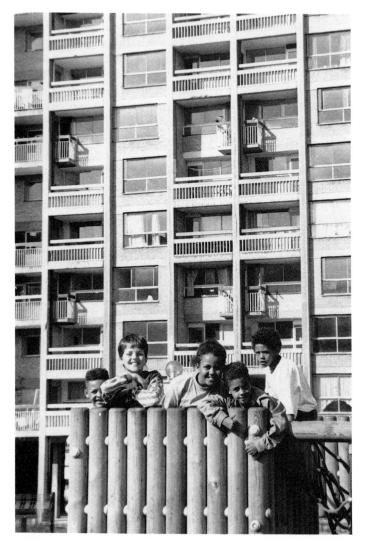

Figure 7

although this is congruent with the enabling and empathic style of practice of the biographical and spiritual aspects of the practitioner, the skills required for these types of action are not those to be found in the conventional general practice. The activity that is generally *called* health promotion in general practice is very often simply prevention (restricted to the personal sphere and the biomedical model), although there is the possibility for practice nurses to take on more responsibility for empowering ongoing groups and ultimately more scope for collective action.

The core values of the practice include accepting responsibility to work to improve the health of the population as well as to provide care and management of disease. This involves making time and resources available for prevention (even though this means reducing the time and resources available for care and disease management) and actively developing collaboration to promote health.

From 'his patient' to 'its population'

It is possible to see at least three ways in which the transition from 'patient' to 'population' has occurred, and a possessive pronoun is retained to indicate that just as doctors have a somewhat proprietorial interest in their patients' interaction with illness, practices have since 1990 accepted a responsibility for their population's health.

Although the population responsibility was originally adopted by pioneering practitioners ('*his* population'), its systematic adoption requires an organizational response by the practice. A population responsibility includes the awareness by the practice of the population as *all the patients* and the choice of the population as an *object of investigation*. While these perspectives may arise from an individually-orientated social philosophy, a collectivistically-orientated social philosophy[31] accepts the population *as an entity* with its own needs, which may coincide with the needs of its individual members or may conflict with them.

The population as *all* the patients

Practitioners may be quite unaware of the needs of those members of their practice population who do not consult or who consult infrequently. When practitioners audit the care they give to particular population groups, they may find that although the patients they know are receiving good care, the patients whom they for some reason do not know are receiving very little. Julian Tudor Hart has described in the UK the 'rule of halves' – half of the patients with raised blood pressure (or non-insulin dependent diabetes mellitus or a range of other conditions) are not detected, half of those detected are not treated and half of those treated are not treated adequately[32].

The practice takes on the core value of making the service available to *all* patients, including responsibility for call and recall systems. It makes use of the gift of the 'list' system of British general practice.

Equity and access

A practice that considers genuinely all its patients will inevitably have to address the question of access to its services. The values of the practitioner involve doing the best in the circumstances, while the values of the practice may involve changing the circumstances. A model based purely on the consultation may, on an individual level, make do with a less than ideal context (eg the absence of an interpreter or advocate or the presence of a doctor of the wrong gender). An organization committed to a population focus can identify barriers to health care, such as language, faced by the population. This may lead to change (eg the employment of an interpreter or more women doctors) to enhance the care given to people within these groups. It is not that some groups of people have 'special' needs because they are homeless, because they are black, because they do not speak English or because they are disabled. They have the same fundamental needs of access to appropriate and acceptable health care as everybody else, but they have real problems in getting their needs met. Meeting the needs of the 'hardest-to-reach' groups can improve services for the whole population (Figure 8).

There is, however, a potential conflict of interest for practitioners and practices about some patients who wish to join a practice list. Some of the most needy people, such as the homeless, are the least likely to be registered with a general practice. This is partly due to the low priority given by the homeless to health care when issues of survival such as food, shelter and income are paramount. However, the system also presents them with additional barriers; for example, general practices require an address for registration. Members of groups such as travellers, refugees, black and minority ethnic people, gay people, women wanting home deliveries and opiate users may feel that general practices discriminate against them on the basis of negative stereotypes or because of the complexity of their social and health needs.

As far back as 1948, GPs collectively accepted responsibility for the whole population of the country and gave the executive councils (and, thus subsequently, health commissions) the power to register patients against the wishes of an individual GP.

The ethics of the practitioner insist that she provide immediate and necessary treatment to any who need it and encourage a tolerant rather than a selective approach to the provision of care in general. A one-to-one consultation is most likely to be satisfactory where it occurs by mutual choice. It is inappropriate for a patient to have to consult a practitioner

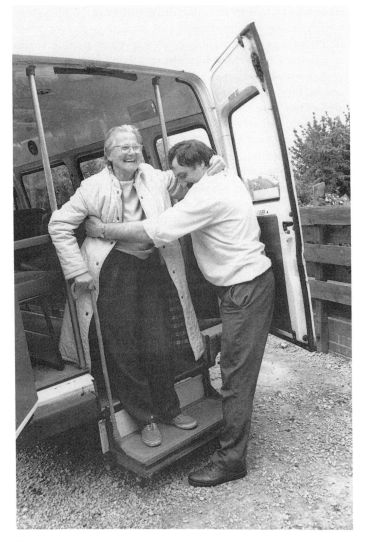

Figure 8

whom she feels unable to trust, and it is similarly less than ideal for a practitioner to have to consult with a patient to whom she feels unable to extend that trust.

> A practice must balance the needs and wishes of individual patients against those of the practice population as a whole. In addition to excluding any patients at the reasonable request of its practitioners (including nurses and receptionists), it may also have to consider excluding patients whose presence is harmful to its other patients. This may occur when an individual patient threatens or expresses violence to other patients in the surgery, but practice values must ensure that this is not used to discriminate against minority or 'difficult' groups.

The FMI initiative, in which budgetary control is devolved to the level of an individual practice, has added a new dimension to these practice decisions whose resolution depends on whether the practice sees its loyalties as limited to the patients currently on its list or to a wider population. A practice will clearly harm the interest of its existing patients if it takes on new patients who either incur greater than average costs or invoke on the practice financial penalties (eg people who choose not to accept cervical smears, blood pressure screening or childhood immunizations). The core values of the practice include responsiveness to its contract with the health commission, and it seems necessary for the commission to clarify whether the practice should limit its responsibility to the registered list or extend it to a defined geographical area.

Follow-up of disease

Who is responsible for the follow-up of disease – the practitioner or the patient? Most practitioners would probably believe that this, like other aspects of diagnosis and treatment, is most properly left to negotiation between the two. Where the patient is unable or unlikely to appreciate fully the importance of follow-up (which may be due, for example, to poor explanation by the practitioner, anxiety or denial in the patient, learning difficulty, mental illness etc), it will be appropriate for the practitioner to take at least some responsibility. In other situations, practitioners know that there is a fine line to be drawn between taking responsibility and creating dependency. Accepting the population responsibility will lead to the practice taking more responsibility for follow-up (away from its patients). If a patient chooses, for example, not to take drug treatment for high blood pressure, the well-meaning efforts of practices to ensure 'compliance' will conflict with that individual's freedom. The other side of this coin is that patients who have come to rely on the annual reminder to attend, for example for a diabetic check, may fail to take adequate responsibility for their own management. Although this may manifest at an organizational level (for example if the patient moves to a practice without a recall system), its most dangerous effect is that it reinforces the belief of some patients in the practitioner's responsibility for their health (for example by prescribing tablets) rather than in their own responsibility (for example their diet).

Prevention of illness for healthier individuals

Practitioners turn naturally to strategies of prevention, which target those at high risk. Strategies of this type identify individuals at high risk (for example of high blood pressure, raised cholesterol, depression or drug abuse) and intervene with this group, while ignoring the rest of the population. Such a strategy 'succours some needy individuals, but the main problem persists'[33]. It is attractive to practitioners because it represents an extension of practitioner values of doing the best possible for the individual, in this case the high-risk individual.

A practice is better able to adopt a 'population' strategy for prevention, to address the risk status of the population as a whole.

Where either strategy involves the practice actively encouraging patients to take up preventive measures, the ethical basis is quite different from that of responding to patients' wishes, whether these be for treatment or prevention. While it is acceptable for a practitioner to do the best possible in response to a patient's wishes, a practice must have absolute confidence that the benefits of its preventive programme outweigh the risks[34].

The population as an object of investigation

Diagnosis

One aspect of the work of a general practitioner is the making of biomedical diagnoses. Some diagnoses may be made by pattern recognition and some by applying a causal approach, but the approach must often involve the weighing up of probabilities[35]. Probabilistic diagnosis requires a knowledge of the prevalence of diseases, signs and symptoms in the population in which the diagnosis is to be made. This knowledge is usually acquired implicitly by the experience of practising in this population but can be made more explicit by direct measurement of these prevalences in the practice population. In this way, epidemiology serves the consultation, rather than vice versa[36].

Health needs assessment

Knowledge of the population also enables health care planners to judge the level of health need in the population as a factor in deciding how much and what health care to commission. One source of information that can contribute to the assessment of health needs is the practice, which requires some assessment of need in order to plan its own services. All practitioners develop an informal knowledge of their populations, but formal studies are required to provide precise measures, particularly where the situation may be changing.

The debate about health needs assessment is still in its infancy, and the involvement of the practice will depend on answers to questions such as:

- What is health?

- Who has the right to determine that something is a health need?

- What balance is to be struck between physical, mental and social health needs?

- What is the best balance between assessing need and facilitating local action?

- What evaluation methods are most appropriate?

Investigation of a population by a practice takes time, and, if no additional funding is provided, the result will be a reduction in time spent by practitioners on other activities, including patient care. Computerized medical records can enable much more efficient retrieval of data, but it is easy to underestimate the time required for the training needed to standardize data input and its coding, as well as to use the data in a meaningful way.

The population as an entity – the public health

It may well be that measures that improve the health of individuals will improve the health of populations and measures that improve the health of populations will improve the health of their individual members. However, there are times when action to improve the health of a whole population will harm some individuals. There are also times when action to improve the health of an individual will reduce the health of the whole population by diverting resources from individuals more responsive to intervention (with greater need).

> The core values appropriate to maintaining the public health are to intervene in the best interests of the population as a whole – in particular, tailoring care and services to objectively measurable need rather than responding to demand – and using the available resources to maximize health gain for the population[37].

Prevention of illness for a healthier population

Immunization has a public health function over and above the protection it gives to individuals. The eradication of smallpox is the most striking example, and the improvement in herd immunity is the explicit aim of many immunization programmes. In this situation, a practice may immunize an individual for the benefit of the population, while any risks of the procedure are borne by the individual. This is usually considered to be compatible with practitioner values, provided there is informed consent and no pressure is applied.

A practice might decide to try to improve the health of its population by reducing the prevalence of obesity, focusing its attention on overweight individuals and exhorting them to lose weight. Even if it succeeds in its population objective, it may simply be adding to the problems of individuals by adding to their sense of guilt. By contrast, a practitioner would be expected to put the needs of the whole patient first, and this might more appropriately take the form of supporting patients in dealing with others who tell them they should lose weight.

Target payments

Public health measures requiring a certain minimum uptake by individuals may only be achieved with a degree of coercion or, at least, persuasion. For example, the coercion for immunization in the USA is handled by the state via the school system and in France via the benefit system.

Although payment for professional services by 'item of service' may be open to abuse through over-provision, practitioners in the 1980s would generally accept parents' wishes not to have their child immunized, provided the risks and benefits had been discussed. Target payments may increase the leverage of 'payment by results' if the practice is close to its target level (or reduce the leverage if the practice is far from its target). This may achieve its objective of increasing immunization uptake and is quite compatible with the values of the practice. If individual practitioners respond to these payments, however, they may find themselves unable truly to empower individual patients to make their own decision. Patients may suspect that they are being advised 'to have their child immunized for the benefit of the population or, indeed, for the benefit of the practice income.

A similar situation can occur when a practice responds to target payments for cervical cytology. When an individual declines to have a smear and the practitioner tries to persuade her to change her mind during the course of consultations carried out for other purposes, the sense of both of them being present for the benefit of the individual patient may be destroyed. The practitioner has been using practice values – putting the public health (reduced incidence and costs of treatment of invasive cervical cancer) before individual freedom.

Rationing

By far the most important conflict between individual and population needs occurs because of the need to ration health care expenditure (prioritize areas of expenditure). Until the last half century, the potential in most science- and technology-driven activities was limited chiefly by technological factors. In 1948, it was a reasonable hope that a comprehensive health care system could deliver high quality care to a whole population, even though the NHS was probably never funded sufficiently to achieve this. It is not unreasonable to imagine that in 1994, even with the breakdown in the post-war consensus in favour of the welfare state, a comprehensive service could be provided if it were limited to the technological interventions available in 1948.

The central questions about health care delivery have changed from 'What can medical science achieve?' to 'What can people afford?'. Because individuals and societies have other claims on their wealth, they may choose not to provide fully for their health needs. Indeed, it is unlikely that in any society the contented[38] will contribute enough, through income redistribution or through health care financing, to ensure that even the most basic needs of all are met.

Rationing of secondary care can be carried out in several ways. Traditionally in the NHS, it was carried out by service planners using a 'command' model. General practice developed in an NHS in which secondary care provision was rationed by waiting lists; these were decided by those planning and financing the service and were partly modified by local variations in cost-effectiveness. An alternative is for secondary care to be rationed by general practice, as agents of the patient, using the supply and demand model of the market economy. In this situation, demand for secondary care is limited by the ability of the patient's agent to pay for it. Fundholding practices now hold a fund with which to purchase a range of secondary care provision and thus act as agents of their patients in expressing demand. To date, this fund has usually been sufficiently generous for fundholders to purchase for their patients at least as good, and sometimes better, secondary care as non-fundholders. If this level of funding is not maintained, it will be general practices that decide which of their patients are treated and which are not. In this situation, the core values of the practice are likely to suggest using the fund in such a way as to achieve the utilitarian goal of the 'greatest good for the greatest number' (probably interpreted as the maximal health gain for the population). The correct decision for the greatest good for some will mean that the practice has to refuse treatment to others of its patients. The values of the practice conflict here with the values of the practitioner.

Rationing of primary care. Practitioners have experience of rationing on the basis of need as they must, for example, decide when to bring a consultation to an end on the grounds that little further benefit is likely from pursuing it, while time might more usefully be spent with another patient. In 1990, the tasks included in the GP's contract were increased, causing a redistribution of resources within the practice that was not just towards population-based and health-based activity but away from individual consultation-based patient care. Many practices tried to avoid this latter aspect by income-generating restructuring (particularly of health promotion clinics) and, indeed, due to departmental underestimation of the number of clinics that would be run, were able to do so in the first year. However, in the medium term, the adoption of a population approach, and a health approach, without an overall increase in resources must lead to a reduction in resources available for individual consultation-based patient care that responds to patients' wants. Care of the population is in conflict with care of the individual, practice values with practitioner values.

Industrial action

To withdraw the provision of medical care from a patient for political reasons is clearly counter to practitioner values. Yet a practice might feel that to take action to publicize the under-funding of the NHS was in the long-term best interests of its patients. Although such a decision may result in a conflict of values, it may also provide an example of the way the values, clearly expressed, can be mutually supportive; during a period of industrial action, the practice may tolerate the practitioner making herself available to any patients who really want a consultation, while the practitioner tolerates the difficulties imposed by the practice.

User and community participation

While the practitioner in the consultation relates to, negotiates with and is accountable to an individual patient, the practice needs to engage with its population, and can do so in a variety of ways:

- to individuals as consumers (a consumerist model)
- to representatives of the population (a democratic model)
- to existing and potential groups within the population (a community development model).

Core values of the practice include formal accountability to users, their representatives and community groups and making alliances for the promotion of health. The consumerist model is exemplified by the Patient's Charter, and the democratic model has not been developed at the practice level. The community development model has included initiatives, such as patient participation groups, that have originated within the practice and various forms of involvement with groups originating outside the practice.

Patient participation in general practice

The early patient participation groups arose from the interest of individual practitioners and began by engaging with the interests of the practitioner. A later development has been user groups whose concerns have been closer to those of the practice. The most important aspect of this form of involvement has been a movement away from a 'them and us' relationship towards an equal partnership[39].

Self-help and community groups

Voluntary sector organizations and community groups can be key players and allies, both in terms of understanding health needs and promoting health. In many instances, they have been established in response to the needs of marginalized groups and can provide support and information. Self-help groups, for example, provide support by sharing experiences of coping with a particular problem or condition in its members' daily lives. In so doing, they play their part in re-establishing autonomy and coming to terms with uncertainty as well as the physical consequences of the condition and its treatment. Working with such groups is compatible with the values of both practitioners and practices, although practices will have greater resources to do so.

Community participation and needs assessment

Clinical assessments of need, of the quality of care and of the effectiveness of medical interventions are of great importance in commissioning health care. However, they do not take into account the experience of health care or the factors that shape that experience, which a user perspective can give. Users have knowledge and experience that can provide essential insights into an understanding of their condition and the impact it has on their lives, as well as the impact of their life circumstances on their health and access to health care. At the planning level, the challenge is to integrate technical needs assessment (which is compatible with practice values) with assessing people's wants. Felt health needs are often very different from those considered as important by public health physicians, often focusing on concerns such as housing, pollution, road safety and access to primary care, rather than cigarette smoking, diet and exercise. Responding to these felt needs may, therefore, run counter to apparent practice values, unless it is committed to a community development approach as meeting these needs may not appear to be the most cost-effective way of maximizing health gain.

Community-orientated primary care

One formal method that practices can use to integrate the personal and population responsibilities (and thus practitioner and practice values) is community-orientated primary care[40]. The method provides a toolkit that a practice can use to share knowledge about the population (drawn from its knowledge of individual patients, from practice records and from information sources outside the practice), to prioritize an area for intervention and to plan, implement and evaluate the intervention. A community-orientated primary care approach provides opportunities for workers in a practice to share concerns about the sometimes conflicting needs of populations and individuals.

From 'the doctor' to 'the practice'

There have been many forces at work encouraging the development of the general practice as an organization. A practice, as a multidisciplinary team, is better able than a practitioner working alone to manage successfully a broader range of health problems, to practise prevention and promotion of health, to take responsibility for the health care of a population as well as its individual members and to gather the data necessary for contract monitoring. The practice is particularly well placed to establish partnerships for health with other organizations (eg welfare rights or community health projects). Practitioners can provide each other with mutual support – physically by sharing on-call duties, mentally by sharing and discussing clinical problems and emotionally by providing immediate support in times of crisis.

In view of all these factors, it may seem surprising that the single-handed practice not only survives but is popular with its patients. Along with the advantages of the larger organization go disadvantages, which for some patients and some practitioners may outweigh the advantages. For practitioners, the disadvantages include the time needed for the communication, meetings and decision-making that are essential to the maintenance of health of the organization. They also include the loss of autonomy and control, both over individual patient management and over the context in which they work, in particular over the levels of practice income (and thus workload) and expenditure (and thus staffing levels and quality of service). This may be no more than the fear that the quality of the organization is only as good as the quality of its weakest link, but a practitioner can come to believe that she is indispensable and be unable to share patient care or even practice decisions. However, for patients and practitioners alike, a central problem with a large general practice is the difficulty of recognizing and being recognized as an individual, the difficulty of receiving and providing continuous personal care.

In this chapter, we will now consider in more depth how the development of the practice has affected the provision of continuous personal care and the boundary with secondary care. We will then look at the ways in which the more general issues of power, ethics and accountability have required redefinition during the development of the practice.

Is personal care compatible with teamwork?

The practitioner

Continuity of care has been identified as a core value of the practitioner. It is not simply the continuity of the medical case record or even the continuity of care in one episode of illness, important as these are. It is, rather, a personal relationship between one practitioner and one patient. The same person may bring one problem today and another one next month or next year. Despite the separation in time, there may be a connection, at the very least, in the way that a person responds to illness, treatment and practitioners. What is done today may have an important bearing on future health. Seeing the same patient for different problems inevitably concentrates interest and attention on the person and his character, story, expectations, family and background. This is the root of the familiarity between two people: mutual understanding and trust that continues to be tested – and usually strengthened – by repeated encounters.

Continuity of personal care can occur most intensely in a single-handed practice, when doctors in group practice have personal lists[41] or when the group of doctors is small. For nurses also, this depends on the number of nurses in the practice and the way they share out the work.

The practitioner's work *looks* easier and more efficient if patients are expected to see whomever is available, and receptionists can keep the queue moving more smoothly if they can fit a patient in with anyone. It saves time if all the visits in one direction on one day are given to the doctor who happens to have to go that way. In any case, the fewer the home visits, the more the economy of time. Off-duty nights and weekends are precious, even if a patient is dying at home and one has known her for a long time. When one does not see the same people regularly, one is not likely to get so emotionally involved in their psychological problems and the pressures which these impose, and patients are less likely to talk about them.

Do patients actually want continuity today? Freeman and Richards[42] have shown that three quarters of patients in their study in Wessex said it was important to see the same doctor each time they visited the practice, and the proportion was even higher in the practice that actually used personal lists. They have also shown that when continuity of care is provided, patients are more likely to discuss a personal problem. The importance of continuity is not universal and depends on the needs and attributes of both practitioners and patients. Continuity is of greater importance for older patients, those with an external health locus of control (a tendency to attribute control of health to fate or the doctor rather than themself) and those with an introvert rather than extrovert personality[43]. Patients clearly vary in the importance they attach to continuity, and even when people generally want continuity, they will at times wish to be able to see a different practitioner, for example because of their gender or special interests, as a second opinion or simply to avoid delay. When anonymity is important, for example when patients fear judgemental attitudes or breaches of confidentiality, continuity of care may be a problem to contend with rather than a value to be defended.

Doctors are, of course, not the only members of the organization to provide continuity. There are many practices, particularly since the departure of doctors as a result of the 1990 contract, in which receptionists and nurses are the longest-established members (Figure 9). The nursing profession has taken seriously the felt need for continuity of care and responded by allocating to each patient a 'named nurse'.

The practice

The practice can provide an additional form of continuity of care, based on the overt commitment of its practitioners to work together in the interests of the patient. The identity of the individual health care worker is probably less important if patients can expect from a practice that they will be recognized and treated as individuals and given time to be heard and to be involved in their own management.

When practitioners adopt a consistent approach and communicate well as a team, they may be trusted and relied upon as a relatively permanent entity, even when personnel change. One sign that the practice has managed successfully to demonstrate this corporate image is hearing patients refer to the practice ('the London Road surgery') rather than the practitioners ('Dr Smith's surgery').

The existence of an organization valuing individuals in this way may feel more important to the patient than a (possibly accidental) personal relationship with one doctor. The continuity of care by practitioner and by practice may be complementary.

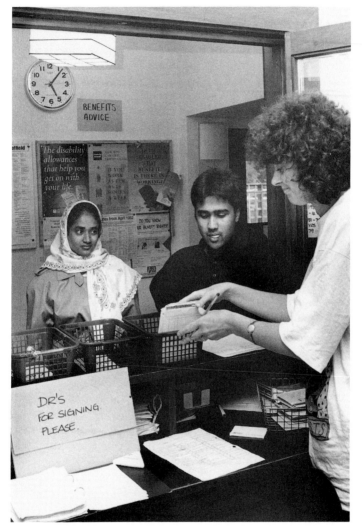

Figure 9

Boundaries with secondary care

The practitioner

The practitioner's relationship with secondary care is an individual professional relationship. The practitioner acts as agent for the patient and takes on the responsibility for referral to an appropriate specialist who is, at best, known to the practitioner and can be expected to provide a quality service. This role in the practice has usually been taken by the doctor, but nurses make increasing numbers of referrals to specialist nurses and (indirectly) doctors.

The practice

As part of the Financial Management Initiative, general practices are increasingly involved in commissioning secondary care, either directly as fundholders or indirectly as commissioning groups advising health commissions. The role and power of managers of fundholding practices and non-fundholding consortia has increased *vis-à-vis* secondary care provider managers.

This commissioning role of the practice strengthens the agency role (in which the practitioner acts as agent of the patient). Also, where the practice relationship builds upon the practitioner relationships, it has the potential significantly to improve the quality of secondary care provided. However, when the practice must consider its financial constraints as a commissioner above the specific secondary care needs of individual patients, the values of the practice are in conflict with the values of its practitioners.

Power

Power, ethics and accountability have different implications for the practitioner and the practice. Power is the ability to make a difference to one's world and may be expressed as 'power over' (power over another) or as 'empowerment' (using power within oneself to enable others to contact the power within themselves). The issue of power in general practice is, at once, central and complex. The model of the practitioner provides one way of clarifying this complexity.

In the caring and biomedical aspects, the practitioner acts to make the patient better and will thus exert 'power over' the patient. The dependency and lack of technical knowledge of the patient is often reinforced by differences in class, gender or race. Patients may collude with this in order to invest their practitioner with the power necessary to defy illness and death on their behalf. In both the biographical and healing aspects, the practitioner sees the patient as a self-healing agent and thus, instead of acting, enables the patient to heal herself. The practitioner thus needs to work in an empowering way.

The practitioner will attempt to integrate these roles. Neither the patriarchal caricature of the biomedical physician nor the consumerist model, with its potential state of conflict between professionals and consumers, is appropriate to the mutual trust desired by both parties. Health and health care are not commodities. They require a power relationship in which, as equal partners, the practitioner can bring knowledge of the general and the patient can bring knowledge of the particular. This form of partnership can enable a patient to make informed decisions and take as much, or as little, responsibility as is appropriate at that time.

The practice, however, often needs to take more 'power over' than does the practitioner. The responsibility of the practice for *health* focuses attention on the prevention of disease and the promotion of health. *Prevention* is a biomedical activity that extends the 'power over' relationship to patients who feel well, in addition to those who feel ill. Promotion of health, on the other hand, should be empowering, although promoting the health of individuals rather than populations can easily take the form of 'power over' by victim blaming.

The responsibility of the whole practice population may be empowering if it leads to removal of blocks to access in service delivery. It can, however, encourage 'power over' when patients are persuaded to use preventive or promotive services they would otherwise not use, when population needs are placed above individual needs (eg herd immunity) and particularly when rationing decisions are made.

This issue of power may illuminate one of the causes of the discomfort felt by GPs in the context of contemporary general practice. They have often chosen to enter general practice because they feel more comfortable with the empowerment inherent in the biographical practitioner than with the 'power over' of the biomedical model in which they were trained. They now find themselves again working in an organization in which the culture of 'power over' is growing.

Ethical systems

The ethical systems required for situations of empowerment differ from those required for situations of 'power over'. Where a practitioner takes 'power over' a patient, this power needs to be tempered by an ethic requiring power to be used solely for the benefit of that patient. This is particularly relevant to the biomedical and caring aspects of the practitioner.

At times, it may not be clear to the practitioner how the 'power over' should be used (eg when it is not known which treatment is most likely to be effective), and a clinical trial may be indicated. At other times, the practitioner may wish to use the relationship for the benefit of others (eg teaching). In both these situations, the patient is invited to give informed consent to increasing the knowledge and skills of biomedical physicians as a group (teaching and research), but this situation must here be completely out in the open.

In situations of empowerment, the purpose of the ethics is principally to ensure that the practitioner does not move into a 'power over' relationship. In particular, in the biographical and healing aspects, practitioners must ensure that they are not unwittingly using the consultation to meet their own needs. This requires them to develop a self-awareness, for example through supervision, of their own emotional responses in the consultation.

Practitioners are able to build up an ethic that is compatible with all these: to act in the interests of the individual patient, take as little 'power over' the patient as is needed, inform and gain consent when 'power over' is necessary. They will also need to care for their own wellbeing so these principles can all be used to the benefit of the patient.

The practice could be considered to require an ethic of acting in the interests of the practice population, taking as little 'power over' the population as is needed, informing and gaining consent when 'power over' is necessary. Care must be taken of the wellbeing of the practice, so that it can be used to the benefit of the practice population.

In spite of the similarity of these two ethics, it seems likely that the practice will always need to exert more 'power over'. In the most extreme case, it is rare for a practitioner to act against the wishes that a patient is expressing; the situations are those in which the practitioner would first consult with a defence body or a court. However, a practice must be prepared to act against the wishes of individuals for the overall benefit of the population. This could produce a direct conflict between practitioner and practice, for example when a practitioner (doctor, nurse or counsellor) defends a patient's individual right to smoke in stressful consultations while the practice attempts to implement its no-smoking policy.

A major advantage of seeing the ethics employed by a practice as different from those of the practitioner is that decisions appropriate to each can be separated out. Practice decisions, such as rationing, can be taken at an organizational level by a group of people making *policy* decisions. Individual practitioners can take part in these decisions (indeed, it is important that the practitioner perspective is heard), but the policy is a practice policy. The practitioner, with awareness, can then return to one-to-one consultations, fully identify with the practitioner values and advise the patient how best to exploit the available possibilities. Even where this change of roles is handled with real self-awareness, however, it is not difficult to imagine the reluctance that practitioners might have in employing the sort of tactics that they are prepared to use to empower patients in their dealings with a health commission (eg letters to MPs or phone calls to the editor of the local paper), when these are directed against the practitioner's own organization and are indeed decisions to which she is party![43]

> *Systems of Survival* by Jane Jacobs[43] is a dialogue on the morality appropriate in the area of work (as opposed to the area of personal morality). She identifies two moral syndromes, each appropriate in its own circumstances.
>
> The 'guardian' syndrome is appropriate where an organization is attempting to act in what it believes to be the best interests of society by taking 'power over', such as defending territory, enforcing the law or ensuring the public health. These actions include those of governments, including the health commission and its agent, the practice.
>
> The 'commercial' syndrome is appropriate where people openly pursue their own self-interest, as in commercial dealings. It is appropriate when there is no taking of 'power over' and includes much of the practitioner role.
>
> Interestingly, Jacobs identifies as destructive situations in which aspects of the two syndromes are mixed or where attempts are made, without due self-awareness, to hold both syndromes simultaneously.

Accountability

The different forms of power and the differing underlying ethics require different forms of accountability, in addition to accountability in law. Both practitioners and practices need to be accountable to patients (or populations), to peers and to commissioners.

Accountability to patients and populations

Practitioners need to be accountable to individual patients. The direct accountability within each consultation is embodied in the principle of informed consent. Where this breaks down, the practitioner is indirectly accountable through the complaints procedure, although the unsatisfactory nature of these procedures for both patients and practitioners is well known[44].

Practices need to be accountable to their population, and thus to individuals and groups within the population, and to the elected representatives for the area. This accountability has, in the past, been poorly developed but is being strengthened by the reforms that have resulted in annual reports and meetings to discuss the changes and by the Patient's Charter, which has clarified consumer rights.

The consumerist view is that it should be as easy to complain about general practice as it is to take a faulty garment back to a chain store. However, consultations are frequently important (in the sense of having long-term implications for health and even life) and personal (in that patient and practitioner need to reveal something of themselves to each other) and in both these ways differ from the purchase of a garment, whose seller is simply passing on in good faith something produced in a factory of which she has no direct knowledge. Complaints about consultations are often of profound personal significance to both practitioner and patient.

Traditionally, practitioners have responded to complaints as individuals. The complaint is likely to be experienced as a complaint about a relationship, about the practitioner as an individual. The practitioner may respond in ways that improve future consultations, but it is also likely that, at least in the short term, these consultations will be impaired by a loss of trust in the patient, loss of self-valuation and a globally impaired ability to tolerate uncertainty.

Practices are much better placed to cope with complaints than are individual practitioners. As organizations, they can minimize the personal significance and importance of a complaint for both patient and practitioner, appreciating the learning experience at an organizational level. Complaints against practitioners reflect their working conditions (eg duration of consultations, work-load and sleep). It may be helpful for complaints to be seen to be directed towards practices rather than towards practitioners.

Accountability to peers

Practitioners see their main channels of accountability as being to their peers. Doctors accept their accountability to the General Medical Council, nurses to the UK Central Council for Nursing. The scope of accountability has widened from 'gross professional misconduct' to less extreme degrees of unfitness to practise. Accountability to peers has been encouraged by the Royal College of General Practitioners. It is probably strongest among training practices and is being strengthened by the increase in clinical audit activity.

One form of clinical accountability is the increasing acceptance by practitioners of the importance that the biomedical care they provide is based on evidence and that one way of achieving this is the use of evidence-based guidelines. These have been more readily accepted by nurses than by doctors. Their value depends crucially on the credibility of the guidelines and the flexibility with which they are applied. Credibility of guidelines requires both that they are firmly based in current evidence and that the recommended actions are appropriate for the population and situation of primary care[45].

Flexibility requires that guidelines are seen as a starting point from which the individual's needs are best met, rather than as a rigid prescription for action – that they are indeed guidelines and not a description of accepted or desirable practice[46]. An intervention that produces the best overall results in a controlled trial may not be the most appropriate for an individual patient (just as it was proved not to be in those patients in the original trial who were withdrawn or who had negative outcomes). For this reason, accountability through guidelines must be accountability to another who can discuss individual patients – accountability to peers rather than to commissioners.

Practices need a broader definition of the term 'peer', one that includes all those working in the practice. This form of accountability of the practice is supported by organizational and interprofessional[47] audit. The development of genuine accountability within the practice, to peers as so defined, is extremely difficult to achieve, as the doctors are the employers of the others, and this difficulty is frequently compounded by differences in class, gender, education and professional status. Some practices are, however, attempting to increase the accountability of doctors by extending the appraisal of staff (by doctors) to include the appraisal of doctors (by staff). There is little likelihood of this accountability becoming strong or widespread until health commissions contract with practices rather than practitioners and the practice becomes the employer.

Accountability to commissioners

Practices see their main channel of accountability as being to the health commission. The practice is particularly aware of the accountability that stretches up the NHS management structure to ministerial level and on to the Treasury. Practice accountability has been greatly increased as commissions have required more data for the purposes of contract monitoring.

As far as practitioners are concerned, GPs are currently directly accountable to the health commission through their terms of service. They may feel the increased financial and managerial accountability that extends into the consultation to be destructive to professional accountability and even to accountability to patients.

The most helpful way of managing this accountability may be for there to be contractual accountability of the practice to the commission[48], with practitioners being accountable directly to the practice and thus only indirectly to the commission.

The general practice and its core values

Having explored the roles and values of the practice under several headings, it is now possible to bring together the different aspects of the practice in a model and to summarize the practice values.

The practice

The practice can usefully be represented by a model similar in outline to that of the practitioner (Figure 10).

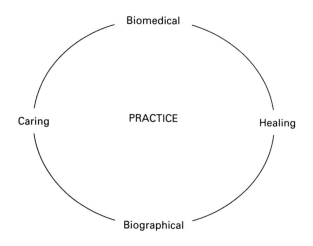

Figure 10

The *biomedical* aspect of the practice, involving predominantly doctors and nurses, can be developed beyond the possibilities available to an individual practitioner. Provision of space and equipment allows more procedures to be carried out with greater quality. Division of labour and specialization can improve quality of care as the knowledge- and skills-base of the practice expands. The application of preventive measures to whole populations can be administered more efficiently and thoroughly. Provision of information and advice (in the form of leaflets, videos, books and advice workers) can be much more extensive.

The *biographical* aspect of the practice can be developed by involving not only doctors and nurses, but also counsellors and psychotherapists. The strength of the practice in this area is particularly clear when working with groups of patients. This may include groups for psychotherapy, support and self-help (eg carers and people suffering with particular chronic illness), local history and reminiscence projects, community art projects (eg theatre, video and visual art). This biographical resource within the practice can also provide some emergency emotional support to practitioners.

The *caring* aspect of the practice can be developed in particular through co-ordination and facilitation, for example of volunteer visitor and transport schemes, advocacy, buddying and befriending schemes, alarm systems, helplines and supporting wholefood co-operatives. There is also a sense in which the caring by all the individuals in the practice results in a caring organization that has an existence in its own right.

The *healing* aspect of the practice is usually the least well developed. To an even greater extent than with the practitioner, the inclusion of this aspect represents a potential rather than a present reality. There is in particular a possibility for the practice to become involved in ceremony – a group of people sharing meditation, yoga or Tai Chi might be an example.

The values

Having described the role of a general practice, it is possible to bring together a provisional list of the core practice values (Table 3.1).

Table 3.1 A summary of practice values

The population: Recognizing the registered practice population as a whole and accepting responsibility for its health and health care
- broader remit, including health
- responsibility to the population of registered patients, whether or not they consult
- fair distribution of resources
- managing the coherence of connections

The practice: Maintaining the quality of the organization
- organizational competence
  - systems, communication
  - contractual responsibility
  - audit (interprofessional)
  - connections with the system
  - developmental capacity (adaptive)
  - managing resource use
- buildings, equipment, appropriate work-load
- safe, supportive environment
- vision/measures of success

The intent: Action in the best interests of the registered practice population
- using available resources to maximize health gain for the population
- equity
- recognizing and overriding conflict of interest between population and practice
  - putting interests of patients before practice finances
- recognizing and overriding conflict of interest between the whole population and individuals
  - tailoring care and services to objectively measurable need rather than demand
- accountability to users/representatives
- accountability to health commissions

Table 3.1 *continued*

- extended proactive role
  – systematic health needs assessment
- systematic prevention/health promotion

The means: Providing, commissioning and alliances
- division of labour, teamwork
- care by the most appropriately skilled
- access by whole practice population
- advocacy for population, rationing
- effectiveness as a key factor
- efficiency as driving force
- information systems, call and recall
- commissioning appropriate secondary care
- 'power over'
- wider alliances for health promotion
- intersectoral (multiagency) working
- political action

Some possible futures 4

This chapter describes some of the possible futures for general practice and the factors that might influence their development. It begins with a consideration of the changing roles within general practice and then looks at the possibility that the generalist role might disappear as a result of present pressures and expectations. The possible consequences of the erosion of the practitioner's core values by the values of the practice are then discussed.

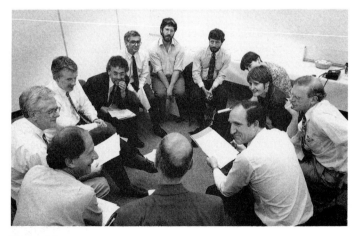

Figure 11

Two possible future contexts for general practice are then considered. In the first, practices exert more 'power over' their patients, health commissions exert more 'power over' practices and the NHS Executive exerts more 'power over' health commissions. In the second, practices are enabled to develop an empowering way of working with communities as well as individuals, as one of many community resources working for health for all (Figure 11).

Changing roles within general practice

Probably the most significant change in the balance of roles within general practice has been the increasingly important part played by non-clinical workers. In the three years following the 1990 contract, the number of practice managers has risen by 43%, that of computer operators by 300% and that of reception, administrative and clerical staff by 29%[49]. Most significant is the increase in number, power and status of practice managers, particularly in fundholding practices, responsible for larger budgets and dealing directly with senior managers in provider units. The number of practice nurses has also risen, by 51%. It has been said that the 1990 contract was not a GP's contract but a practice nurse and practice manager contract.

Practitioners may feel increasingly the need to choose between traditional values of the practitioner and the increasingly dominant values of the practice. Since the 1990 contract, GPs may have tended to carry on much as before, expecting practice managers and nurses to take on new functions and values[50]. In many fundholding practices, a single enthusiastic doctor has identified with 'the practice' and led it into fundholding, while the other partners have acquiesced or involved themselves only in the aspects that were congruent with their existing values (eg collaboration with colleagues about rational prescribing and referral guidelines).

- One possibility for the future is separation into clinical generalists who function as traditional GPs, and doctors who identify with the dominant culture of the practice and are involved with fundholding, management, data collection, population medicine, health promotion and, perhaps, specialized medical care. It may be possible, particularly with an understanding of the two value systems and the potential for conflict, for an individual to spend some sessions in each role. Many GPs want to identify with both practitioner and practice values. Although this appears to be possible at present it may, with full self-awareness, be a position that is increasingly difficult to sustain, as resources shrink and practitioners have to take responsibility for rationing.

- Another possibility is that generalists may develop their biomedical aspect and shed their caring, biographical and healing roles. This might lead to their development into 'generalists with a special interest', with a purely biomedical role.

- Individuals might, alternatively, choose to leave the generalist role and develop one of their other aspects (caring, healing or biographical), for example retraining as a psychotherapist.

- Practitioners who wish to remain generalists and avoid the practitioner/practice conflict may find it more satisfactory to do this outside the NHS, by working abroad or in private practice.

Practice nurses may also separate into two groups, although they may find it easier than doctors to hold the different sets of values in balance, at least while the majority of their consultations have a focus on health rather than disease.

The practitioner values, being at times in conflict with practice values, are likely at best to be tolerated rather than supported by the practice. The generalist may, therefore, have a rather lower status in the practice than at present, a price to be paid for being accepted within the organization. This raises the question of whether we need this role and, if so, who will take it on. The main primary health care worker in this country has traditionally been medically qualified, but this is not inevitable. The position could, as in less-developed countries, be filled by a nurse. Impetus for such a change could come from several possible sources.

- Nurses already practise as clinical generalists, and many are interested in developing the role beyond its current boundaries. One path is to develop areas of special expertise, such as asthma or diabetes; another is to develop a generalist role as nurse practitioner working alongside or in place of a medically qualified generalist.

- Doctors may decide to leave an undervalued generalist role. One role of a profession is to protect and monopolize knowledge-base, and once this knowledge-base is no longer monopolized or valued, the profession is likely to respond by delegation 'downwards'.

- The Treasury has already stimulated re-examination of skill-mix among nursing teams, and it has been argued that this should be extended to include the whole general practice[51].

- Patients have had increasing opportunity to consult nurses in general practice since the 1990 contract. Some have found it easier to communicate with nurses, who make more time available to them.

In spite of the possibility of change, it seems most likely that doctors will retain a major generalist role, although nurses will develop this aspect of their work. Nurses are likely to experience the same tension as doctors between their role as practitioner and their role in prevention and population medicine.

The disappearing generalist

Anxiety about the disappearance of the old type of family doctor can be traced back at least as far as the 1850s[52]. The generalist role is clearly resilient, but its future is not guaranteed. It may be threatened by the changing expectations of patients, the Treasury and practitioners themselves.

Expectations of the patient

Why wait?

In single-handed practice, particularly in remote rural locations, the doctor's life is visible, and out-of-hours consultations may be delayed until a time convenient to the doctor. As society comes to expect 24-hour availability of a wide range of goods and services, there is pressure in general practice to follow suit[53]. This would result in a rota or shift system of working and thus reduce continuity of care.

Why tolerate uncertainty?

As people take more control over their lives, they may be less willing to tolerate uncertainty. Complaints are more likely to be directed at errors of omission than of commission. Patients may choose increasingly to see a specialist, as they can appreciate the disadvantages of tolerating uncertainty more readily than its advantages (of reducing risk and cost). With the greater availability of information about medical care, including the development of expert systems and self-directed treatment[54], patients may feel they have sufficient knowledge not to need a generalist opinion but to be able to deal with straightforward problems themselves and to select their own specialists appropriately.

Expectations of the Treasury

Measurable inputs, measurable outputs and efficiency

The FMI model (*see* Chapter 3) requires a public service to have measurable inputs and outputs. The measurable outputs of the generalist are either inappropriate to practitioner values (eg patient throughput and referral rates) or difficult to quantify, while the outputs of the practice (eg population targets) are relatively easy to measure. Purchasers find it easier to relate to the inputs and outputs of the practice than of the practitioner. The very process of measuring outputs will direct attention and resources away from practitioners and thus care provided by generalists.

As the Treasury seeks to reduce the costs of health care, it may seek to externalize costs currently borne within the NHS by making patients bear the cost. Home and night visits are expensive, and it may be cheaper for these to be provided in emergency centres (staffed by practitioners working shifts), with patients paying for transport. Although it is quite possible to practise as a generalist without visiting patients' homes, home visits (particularly for emergencies) often make it easier for a practitioner to assess psychosocial factors, and the experience shared by doctor and patient of an emergency visit at night may provide a sound basis for future biographical practice.

If the financial value (in reduced referral, investigation and treatment) of the general practitioner is not appreciated because it is difficult to measure, the Treasury may simply decide that it does not need to purchase a generalist service of any sort. Alternatively, it might choose to purchase a biomedical generalist service with measurable outputs but without any biographical, caring or healing aspects. This could result from a range of attitudes, including a failure to value these aspects, a belief that patients should pay for them directly or a belief that they can be more cheaply or effectively provided by specialists (in caring, healing and biographical practice) than by generalists. More evidence is urgently needed on the cost-effectiveness of primary health care provision by generalists compared with specialists.

Expectations of the practitioner

The security of specialism

There is a great deal of satisfaction and sense of security in developing a special expertise in one field of biomedical expertise. This can enable a 'generalist with an interest in . . .' to compensate for dissatisfaction and insecurity in the generalist role. It has the danger, however, of undermining the generalist skills of colleagues within the same general practice.

Personal safety and comfort

As the interpersonal relationship between doctor and patient weakens, the importance to the doctor of her safety and comfort becomes more important. As the general level of violence in society rises and people put less value on their relationship with their GPs, there is an increasing risk of harm from patients, and GPs feel particularly vulnerable when making home visits[55]. These trends can only reduce the readiness of GPs to make home visits and thus undermine the generalist role.

The health commission, its provider organizations and contracting for health

What of the context within which general practice continues to change? It is possible to describe this context in a way similar to that used for the practitioner and the practice – 'the health commission, its provider organizations and contracting for health'.

Although primary health care is at present commissioned at a national level, it seems likely that an increasing component will be commissioned locally. The strength of this scenario lies in the responsibility of a health commission for the health care of everybody in its geographical area. It is in a position to address issues of equity and access in this area. General practice is thus seen by the commission as one of a number of possible provider organizations. If health commissions enter into contracts with provider organizations, and practitioners contract with these organizations, practitioners can more easily make a choice between the practitioner and the practice values, rather than having to embrace both.

One danger of this scenario is that health commissions may commission care that, while maximizing health gain within the available resources, progressively reduces the time available for those aspects of practitioner care that do not have easily measurable outputs, thereby further weakening practitioner values.

Another danger of this scenario is that it represents 'power over' the providers by the health commission. Since the 1990 contract, FHSAs/health commissions have taken an increasingly active role in the collection of information, the re-allocation of resources between practices and even the content of clinical consultations (eg approval of clinical protocols for chronic disease management). 'Contracts', in the context of a single (monopsonist) purchaser and multiple providers, are not an agreement mutually entered but an instrument for exerting control. Providers will need either to accept this control or to improve their negotiating position. If the power of the health commission to negotiate local contracts is developed, one possible response by practices would be the formation of large provider alliances having local monopolies.

The Financial Management Initiative (FMI) aims to devolve budgetary responsibility (the root of rationing by the practice and thus the most serious point of practitioner/practice conflict) but increase the power of the centre. The centralization of power has been achieved both by increased managerial accountability and by the final removal of any local democratic accountability of the NHS (local authority representatives on health authorities and family practitioner committees)[56], and its replacement by 'consultation' with consumers. The Functions and Manpower Review is likely to result in changes that increase the clarity and directness of the accountability of the health commissions to the NHS Executive and thus to ministers. 'The health commission, its providers and contracting for health' describes a scenario in which government is in a position increasingly to control the content of the consultation and values of the practitioners. It is arguable whether this is a desirable or even (in view of the rapidly changing political priorities) an effective way of managing a health service.

Communities, their enablers and health for all

There is an alternative future, in which there is greater *local* accountability, an enabling power structure and alliances that extend beyond the health care system to promote health at all levels, from local to national. The scenario described by 'communities, their enablers and health for all' puts communities first.

While the NHS was a centrally planned organization, it could be argued that it was appropriate for its accountability to be at a national level. Now that the service is provided by a managed market and responsibility has been devolved, it is appropriate that accountability also be devolved. There are a number of possible mechanisms.

- The *democratic model* could be restored and extended, for example by placing health commissions under the control of local government or by opening health commissions to direct elections.

- The *consumerist model* could be taken to its logical conclusion. Purchasers could be made accountable to patients, using the same market mechanism by which providers are accountable to purchasers. This would involve removing the monopoly position of health commissions, by giving patients the right to choose the health commission that would purchase their health care, irrespective of where they live. A disadvantage of this strategy would be some loss of the ability of the health commission to purchase on the basis of the health needs of the geographical area (although this ability is, anyway, increasingly threatened by further extension of fundholding).

- The *franchise model* is an alternative way of dealing with a natural monopoly and would introduce accountability without altering the geographical responsibility of the commission. In this model, the government grants a franchise monopoly for a fixed length of time to a health commission on the basis of competitive tendering or contestability, thereby opening up the commissioning role to competitive forces[57]. A central question is 'Who would be responsible for awarding the franchise (would it be the chairperson and non-executive directors, the local authority or a new organization attempting, by its membership, to balance the interest of central and local government, patients and providers)?'

In this scenario, the health commission would take on primarily an enabling role. It would have the specific brief of establishing local health needs, commissioning appropriate health care and empowering its providers to respond to local communities of interest among users of the health care service. This enabling role and the establishment of local accountability might (or might not) ensure that people's want for practitioner care would be met. The health commission's role in maximizing health gain for the population would be achieved in part through its provider organizations, with their practice values, and in part by working with other agents responsible for promoting health, such as local authorities, community development projects and community groups.

Central government's role would be one not of detailed monitoring of the service but of setting a strategic direction that takes account of the strengths of existing provision, providing adequate funding and auditing the use of those funds and tackling, at a national level, factors that affect the health of the whole population. Achievement of the Health of the Nation targets, for example, depends more on the Treasury and the Departments of Social Security, Employment, and Transport than on the Department of Health. The result could be better Health for All.

Practitioners and practices – conflicting values

Since 1990, general practice has changed the colour of its skin, like a chameleon, with managers, nurses and some doctors adopting practice values outside the consultation but most retaining their practitioner values within the consultation. If resource levels in general practice were infinite, or even adequate, it might be possible simultaneously to hold practice and practitioner values without significant conflict. This may be the situation in some well-resourced practices at present, but the more general experience has been one of strain[58].

The analogy with the chameleon is based on this animal's ability to change colour so that it does not make itself vulnerable by standing out from its environment. Interestingly, the chameleon's ability to do so is limited, and its most striking colour changes reflect its emotions, particularly fear and anger.

For the majority of practices there are three possible ways of dealing with these conflicts of values:

1 The differences may continue not to be named. The situation continues in which different values are held by different members of the practice, or even the same person at different times, without clarity about what is happening. This approach puts individuals under considerable stress and has the potential for continuing misunderstanding and conflict within the practice (Figure 12).

2 The values of either the practitioner or the practice may attempt to 'colonize' and replace the others.

If practitioner values gain dominance, other than by practitioners working outside the NHS, these practices will fail to develop a full range of services for their patients and fail to play their part in maximizing the health gain of the practice population. These practices are likely to have a troubled relationship with their health commission. Where levels of resource are insufficient for the basic needs of patients to be met (eg where patients feel that practices are rationing their access to care), this may be the only – even partially satisfactory – way for practitioners to cope. In this situation, the health commissions would be driven to take upon themselves the aspects of the practice values that were delegated to practices by the NHS reforms.

If practice values gain dominance, their patients will lose the continuity of personal care that has characterized British general practice and risk losing the biographical, caring and healing aspects of the practitioner and even the very existence of the clinical generalist. These practices are likely to have a troubled relationship with their patients, and those who are financially able to do so may seek their medical care outside the NHS and even outside the bio-medical approach.

3 People may recognize that it is quite appropriate for practitioners and practices to have different core values.

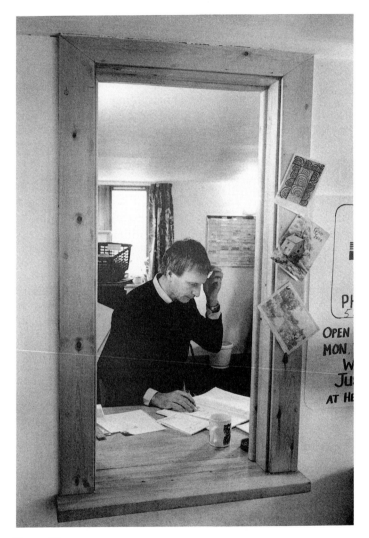

Figure 12

The practice needs values that enable it to manage the contract, ration care and maximize health gain for the whole population within the available resources. It recognizes that it can best achieve these objectives by accepting practitioners who employ in consultations a rather different set of values.

The practitioner needs values that enable her to respond to whatever problems the patient brings, recognizing that there is potential to provide a higher quality service working within a practice that uses different values.

If the third way is to be chosen there are three requirements:

- *Awareness*: If we can be aware of the core values of the practitioner *and* of the practice, we can then nurture them. Where the two sets of core values differ, we can acknowledge the need for the differences without feeling that one set is universally 'right' and the other universally 'wrong'.

- *Appreciation*: We need to respect the equity, population coverage, health dimension and breadth of remit of the practice and find ways of celebrating these, probably together with our patients. We need to respect the values of the practitioner and find ways of celebrating these, perhaps in books and photographs and on video. If the consultation is seen as sacred, there is a need to go into the 'holy of holies', to describe and measure what is happening there and to share it with those who do not already have the experience or share the core values.

- *Action*: Practitioners and practices must not only identify when their core values are not being honoured, but must also take action to bring day-to-day activity into line with core values. This may be most effectively achieved by sharing the core values consciously with patients and inviting them to identify failures in a constructive way. It may be possible for one individual to hold both sets of values at different times of the day, but it may be appropriate for any one person to identify clearly with only one set of values.

If health commissions were to contract with practices rather than practitioners, all of those working in the practice could draw a salary from the practice, perhaps on a profit-sharing basis. This would facilitate the development of a flexible management style and corporate identity. Above all, it would allow practitioners to be clear about the boundaries between practitioner and practice roles and values.

The tension between practice and practitioner values should not be underestimated. The value system of the health commission is closer to those of the practice than the practitioner, and this will influence the conflict between the sets of values within a general practice, risking the under-valuation or even exclusion of practitioner values.

There are other examples of organizations that have diversified, expanded and lost touch with their core. I have recently left the bank I have had my account with for 25 years. This was not because of the barrage of customer satisfaction surveys and relentless offers of financial health checks. It was not even the errors in my current account or the incompletely answered letters. It was the combination of these events that led me to realize that what I saw as the bank's core value, of efficiently handling my money, had been replaced by the values of an insurance broker. Both sets of values are valid, but the old values appeared to have been colonized by the new.

Conclusion

General practices have developed core values (practice values) that differ from those of the doctors, nurses and other workers who have one-to-one involvement with patients (practitioner values).

- *Practitioner* values are appropriate to an individual practitioner whose focus is on the central importance of the individual patient.

- *Practice* values are appropriate to an organization whose focus is on the health of a population. Here the practice's role is to maximize health gain with the available resources.

As we have seen, practitioner and practice values can be mutually reinforcing, but there are areas of conflict, particularly relating to continuity of care and rationing (of both primary and secondary care).

Many practitioners are at present trying to honour both sets of values simultaneously, without always acknowledging the areas of conflict. Practitioners may feel more comfortable and work more effectively if they choose to identify with *either* the practitioner *or* the practice roles and values. This could be facilitated by health commissions contracting with general practices rather than general practitioners. Practitioner values may be more likely to be preserved in a more locally accountable NHS, as they are valued by patients.

Whatever the future configuration of primary health care, the general conclusion reached by this series of King's Fund Capital Conferences is that the core values of both practitioners and practices are of central importance. We need to identify both sets of values and find ways of building on the strengths of each in order to realize the full potential of primary health care.

References

1   Macdonald JJ (1993) Primary health care – medicine in its place. Earthscan.

2   Smith R (1989) Dealing with sickness and incompetence: success and failure. *BMJ.* **298**: 1695–8.

3   Handysides S (1994) Morale in general practice: is change the problem or the solution? *BMJ.* **308**: 32–4.

4   Stott N (1994) The new general practitioner? *Br J Gen Pract.* **44**: 2–3.

5   RCGP Working party (1972) *The future general practitioner. Learning and teaching. BMJ* for RCGP, London.

6   Leeuwenhorst Working Party (1977) The work of the general practitioner. *J Roy Coll Gen Pract.* **27**: 117.

7   Heath I (1993) The future of general practice. In Lock S (ed.) *Eighty-five not out.* pp. 19–22. King's Fund, London.

8   Marinker M (1989) *General practice and the new contract.* In *Greening the White Paper.* Social Market Foundation, London.

9   Moore GT (1992) The disappearing generalist. *The Milbank Quarterly.* **70** (2): 361–79.

10 Oh VMS (1994) The placebo effect – can we use it better? *BMJ.* **309**: 69–70.

11 Balint M (1957) *The doctor, his patient and the illness.* Pitman Medical, London.

12 Charlton BG (1991) Stories of sickness. *Br J Gen Pract.* **41**: 222–3.

13 Huygen FJA (1983) *Family medicine, the medical life histories of families.* Bunner/Mazel.

14 Berger J and Mohr J (1967) *A fortunate man, the story of a country doctor.* Penguin; reprinted 1976 by the Writers and Readers Cooperative, London.

15 Widgery D (1991) *Some lives!* Simon and Schuster, London.

16 Chambers R and Belcher J (1993) Work patterns of general practitioners before and after the introduction of the 1990 contract. *Br J Gen Pract.* **43**: 410–12.

17 Hannay D, Usherwood T and Platts M (1992) Workload of general practitioners before and after the new contract. *Br J Gen Pract.* **304**: 615–18.

18 Co-operative inquiry group (1985) *Whole person medicine: A Co-operative inquiry.* British Postgraduate Medical Foundation, London.

19 Aldridge D (1991) Spirituality, healing and medicine. *Br J Gen Pract.* **41**: 425–7.

20 Rooley A (1990) *Performance – Revealing the Orpheus Within.* Element Books, Shaftesbury, Dorset.

21 Hoggett P (1987) *Why being 'good enough' is good enough*. School for Advanced Urban Studies, Bristol.

22 Huntington J (1992) Ten years – the headlines *Health Service Journal*. **102**: 21.

23 BMA (1965) A Charter for the Family Doctor. *BMJ*. Supplement 89.

24 RCGP working party (1981) Health and prevention in primary care. *Reports from General Practice, RCGP*. **18**. London.

25 Field R (1992) *From rhetoric to reality – teamwork in primary health care*. Report to the Department of Health.

26 Laughlin R and Broadbent J (1994) The managerial reforms of health and education in the UK: value for money or devaluing process? *The Political Quarterly*. **65**: 152–67.

27 Fraser RC, McKinley RK and Mulholland H (1994) Consultation competence in general practice: testing the reliability of the Leicester assessment package. *Br J Gen Pract*. **44**: 293–6.

28 Gorz A (1989) *Critique of economic reason* (translated by Handyside G and Turner C). Verso, London.

29 Housden E and Ford J (1991) General practitioner's pay. *BMJ*. **303**: 1086.

30 Fisher K and Collins J (1993) Homelessness, Health Care and Welfare Provision. Routledge, London.

31 Nijhuis HGJ and Van der Marsen LJG (1994) The philosophical foundations of public health: an invitation for debate. *J Epidemiol*. **48**: 1–3.

32 Hart JT (1988) *A new kind of doctor*. Merlin Press, London.

33   Rose G (1993) Preventive strategy and general practice. *Br J Gen Pract.* **43**: 138–9.

34   Holland WW (1993) Screening: reasons to be cautious. *BMJ.* **306**: 1222–3.

35   Wulff HR (1976) *Rational diagnosis and treatment.* Blackwell Scientific Publications, Oxford.

36   Hodgkin P (1993) Accountants, populations and protocols: reintegrating the diverging mythologies of general practice. Personal communication.

37   Secretary of State for Health (1992) *The health of the nation: a strategy for health in England.* HMSO, London.

38   Galbraith JK (1992) *The culture of contentment.* Sinclair-Stevenson, London.

39   Pietroni P and Chase HD (1993) Partners or partisans? Patient participation at Marylebone Health Centre. *Br J Gen Pract.* **43**: 341–9.

40   Gillam S, Plamping D, McClenahan J, Harries J and Epstein L (1994) *Community orientated primary care.* King's Fund, London.

41   Pereira Gray DJ (1979) The key to personal care. *J Roy Coll Gen Pract.* **29**: 666–78.

42   Freeman GK and Richards SC (1993) Is personal continuity of care compatible with a free choice of doctor? Patients' views on seeing the same doctor. *Br J Gen Pract.* **43**: 493–7.

43   Jacobs J (1992) *Systems of survival: A dialogue on the moral foundations of commerce and politics.* Hodder and Stoughton, London.

44   Donald AG (1993) Quis custodiet ipsos custodes? *Br J Gen Pract.* **43**: 270.

45 Grol R (1993) Development of guidelines for general practice care. *Br J Gen Pract.* **43**: 146–51.

46 McCormick J (1994) The place of judgement in medicine. *Br J Gen Pract.* **44**: 50–1.

47 Clinical Outcomes Group Primary Care Clinical Audit Working Group (1993) *Clinical audit in primary health care.* Department of Health consultation paper. DoH, London.

48 Irvine D (1993) General practice in the 1990s: a personal view of future developments. *Br J Gen Pract.* **43**: 121–5.

49 Department of Health (1994) *Statistics for general medical practice in England and Wales 1994.* Bulletin.

50 Laughlin R, Broadbent J and Willig-Atherton H (1994) Recent financial and administrative changes in GP practices in the UK: initial experiences and effects. *Accounting, Auditing and Accountability Journal.* **7** (3): 96–124.

51 Maynard A and Walker A (1993) *Planning the medical workforce. Struggling out of the time-warp.* Discussion paper 105, Centre for Health Economics, York.

52 Loudon I (1986) Medical Care and the General Practitioner. Clarendon Press, Oxford.

53 Salisbury C (1993) Visiting through the night. *BMJ.* **306**: 762–4, 1750–1850.

54 Troop N, Treasure J and Schmidt U (1993) From specialist care to self-directed treatment. *BMJ.* **307**: 577–8.

55 Hobbs FDR (1991) Violence in general practice: a survey of general practitioners' views. *BMJ.* **302**: 329–32.

56 Pollock AM (1992) Local voices. *BMJ.* **305**: 535–6.

57 Ham C (1994) *Management and Competition in the New NHS.* Radcliffe Medical Press, Oxford.

58 Stott NCH (1993) When something is good, more of the same is not necessarily better. William Pickles lecture. *Br J Gen Pract.* **43**: 254–8.

Index